General
Osteopathic
Treatment

AN INTRODUCTION TO THE PRINCIPLES OF CLASSICAL OSTEOPATHIC TREATMENT

ROBERT JOHNSTON
The Canadian Academy of Osteopathy

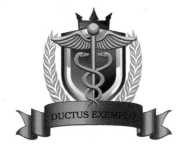

DUCTUS EXEMPLO

With Assistance from
Samuel Jarman & Tana Shepherd

Illustrated by
Jennifer Herring

General Osteopathic Treatment
Copyright © 2015 CAO Press

Robert D. Johnston
With assistance from Samuel Jarman & Tana Shepherd

ISBN: 978-0-9949471-0-9

Canadian Academy of Osteopathy Press
The Canadian Academy of Osteopathy
66 Ottawa Street North
Hamilton, Ontario, L8H 3Z1

Formatted and illustrated by Jennifer Herring
Images modelled by Leah Ryerse and Leah Heney
Cover & chapter dividers designed by Jennifer Herring
Copyediting & publishing consultation by Dr. Jeffrey Douglas

TABLE OF CONTENTS

Please note that due to anatomical variations, the reader may find slight differences between the anatomy illustrated here and other sources. The purpose of the following information is to inspire the reader to approach the human body with an osteopathic mindset in order to investigate the relationships between anatomical functions.

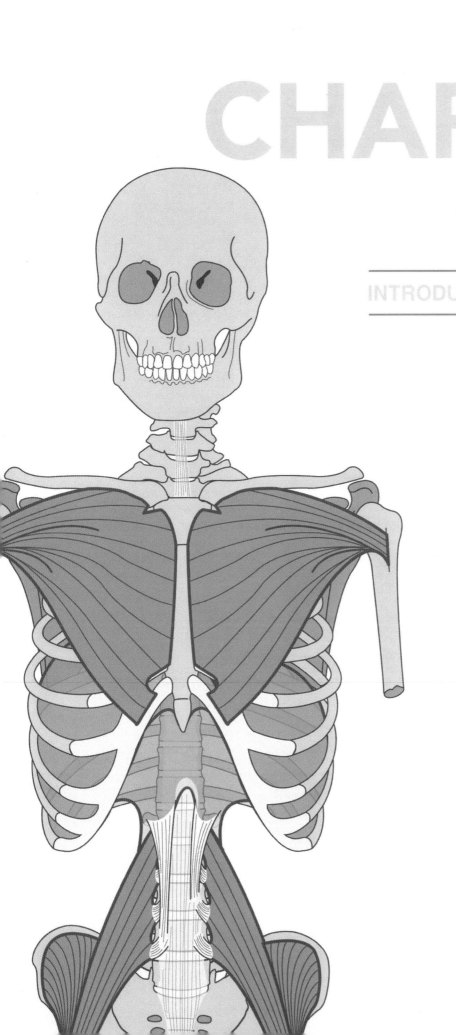

CHAPTER ONE

INTRODUCTORY DISCUSSIONS

Notice to the Reader

The Canadian Academy of Osteopathy provides *classical* osteopathic education based on the concepts and principles established by the founder of Osteopathy—the original Osteopath—Dr. Andrew Taylor Still. The term 'classical', in this case, is used to describe past osteopathic practice as performed in Kirksville, Missouri, by A.T. Still and his earliest students until approximately 1910, a practice that has since changed immensely worldwide. One of the educational goals of the CAO is to investigate the techniques of Dr. Still and his earliest graduates to identify commonalities—what we will hereafter refer to as *Stillian* principles—and pass these methods on to our students so that they can practice classical Osteopathy in its purest form.

Classical Osteopathy was founded on a thorough understanding of the relationship between structure and function; it is based entirely on an exceptional knowledge of anatomy and physiology rather than on the memorization of techniques. As such, classical Osteopathy agrees with any expression of Osteopathy that is likewise grounded in the principles of Dr. Still's understanding of his discovery.

The purpose of generating this handbook is to offer students a comprehensive yet foundational approach to the primary areas through which Osteopathy addresses human physiology. Certain examples concerning the application of technique, therefore, are illustrated in this handbook; however, this text is not intended to be taken as a 'recipe book' for the delivery of osteopathic treatment. The author hopes to give general guidelines for the student, but will refrain from providing specific rules. Once *rules* are prescribed to treatment, the *art* of Osteopathy becomes little more than rigid techniques. The descriptions in this text are a series of isolated scenarios not intended to be taken as limiting, but rather as exemplars from which infinite possibilities and directions might be interpreted.

The essence of osteopathic education is to understand the fundamental, undebatable principles if the reader aims to deliver safe, effective, and efficient osteopathic treatment. These principles encompass the operator's approach (handling, rhythm, and transitions, for example). In other words, this book does not focus on techniques themselves, but rather the principles governing technique. For that reason, all of the examples in the following handbook describe concepts such as the operator's body mechanics, stances, contact and control with the patient, vectoring of force, intention, palpation of the barrier, positioning of the fulcrum, and connecting the lever to that fulcrum. These elements are crucial for the successful delivery of osteopathic treatment; they are the fine points that make all 'techniques' safe, effective, and efficient.

Only after the operator has mastered these principles, and has acquired a full understanding of physiology, can he or she begin to administer successful treatments based on fundamental osteopathic skills. In fact, it is the additional educational goal of the Canadian Academy of Osteopathy to have the student master these principles in such a way that there will be no need for subsequent training on 'technique'. Classical osteopathic education should provide an understanding of the concepts and principles of treatment so thoroughly that Osteopaths are given the freedom to think and apply the principles in their own way.

For this reason, the chapters that follow should be regarded as a starting point. The handbook provides the reader with a reference, in conjunction with classroom material, that complements the introductory stages of their education while they are building the fundamental skills. It is our hope that this book will give students an additional avenue to build their confidence and enhance their table work. Over the next four years of their education, students should be progressively building their technical skill sets so that they can then develop their own approaches, and thus develop into their ideal of a classical Osteopath.

Classical Osteopathy and Osteopathic Thinking

The doctor of the future will give no medicine but will interest his patients in the care of the human frame, in a proper diet, and in the cause and prevention of disease.

—Thomas Edison

Early American classical Osteopathy is founded on the principles of natural law. In the opening of this handbook, then, it is appropriate that the first chapter begin with a discussion of *principles*.

A principle, in familiar terminology, can be succinctly described as:

A comprehensive and fundamental law, doctrine, or assumption; a rule; the laws or facts of nature underlying the working of an artificial device. (*Merriam-Webster*, 2014)

In layman's terms, principles are the laws or states by which something is governed. The world around us is governed by the principle of natural law; the force of an object is dictated by the relationship between its mass and the gravitational pull applied to it; the motion of substances is predictable based on their concentration as well as space allotted to them; and even structures are designed in a way to perform a specific function, such as in tensile strength or aerodynamics. These concepts are all physical principles, components of natural law, that govern the world around us, and they are, of course, as true to that world as they are to the human body.

Natural law is the indisputable theory or principle that governs our world and is thus the foundation of classical Osteopathy. Classical Osteopathy is sometimes, unfortunately, regarded as *old, outdated, or obsolete*. These misconceptions imply that it is the time frame in which Osteopathy was discovered that makes it classical rather than its foundational principles. Of course, *classical* Osteopathy wasn't *classical* in the earliest days of Osteopathy. It was just Osteopathy. What made it *classical* was that it was based upon the science of natural law (anatomy and physiology) that was available to physicians of the time. This approach is no different than the approach taken by the CAO in the classical Osteopathic movement today: we apply today's scientific knowledge, along with the principles of the self-healing and self-regulating mechanisms of the body, to treatment. This approach is as true today as it was in the earliest days of Osteopathy, in the time of Dr. Andrew Taylor Still.

Perhaps the reason classical Osteopathy invites these misconceptions is because some are quick to equate a principles-based approach with stagnation and rigidity. Classical Osteopathy, however, is *progressive* rather than *regressive,* meaning it requires the thinking Osteopath to have a firm, logical foundation that also challenges preconceived notions. This is why it is extremely difficult to teach, to write a book, or to lecture on Osteopathy itself because it necessitates an evolutionary process of thinking. It relies on an impeccable understanding of natural law, on the structure and function of relationships, and belief in the self-healing and self-regulating mechanisms of the human body. Only when these concepts are appreciated can clinicians apply their osteopathic thinking.

As with any scientific advancement, Dr. Still should indeed be credited for the discovery of Osteopathy, as well as for the tenacity with which he laid the first stone in the foundation of the practice. He should be duly credited, not so much as the creator or inventor (for something that is based on natural law cannot be created or invented), but for its unearthing. With his naturalistic approach to health, belief in progression and advancement, and encouragement of spirituality, it's no wonder that he was the founder of the osteopathic profession.

But classical Osteopathy isn't merely the writings of one man. It is not an opinion, as scientific discovery must be based on fact—fact which is, in our case, the logical study of applied mechanics, anatomy, and physiology—and the science of evolving those studies. In the *Autobiography of A.T. Still* (1897), Still writes:

> On June 22nd, 1874, I flung to the breeze the banner of Osteopathy. For twenty-three years it has withstood the storms, cyclones, and blizzards of opposition. Her threads are stronger today than when the banner was first woven. (46)

Although this day marked a significant milestone for Osteopathy, it represented merely the beginning of an ever-evolving approach to treating the human body. While founded on principles, classical Osteopathy, like any other scientific study, requires advancement; thus, there must be a constant evolution of Osteopathy that parallels our scientific understanding in relation to human thought. Dr. Still himself showed progression in his thought process: shortly after his announcement about the discovery of Osteopathy in 1874, he modified his title from 'magnetic healer' to 'bone setter' in 1883, when he was treating in Kirksville, Missouri (Trowbridge, 136). This transition indicated a shift from the mysticism of magnetism (something rife with obscurity because we cannot empirically observe the phenomenon) to bone setting (something tangible and rooted in the structure of causal relationships).

Studying Still's works is of the utmost importance if one wishes to gain an understanding of the principles of natural law, but it does not advocate for the rejection of current scientific study. We have to honour his instructions to 'dig on' (Still, *Personal Papers*). To maintain this classical, principles-based Osteopathy, we must be constantly evolving our thinking while maintaining a firm connection to the science that we have available to us now. The idea of evolution is not *contrary* to classical, principles-based Osteopathy, but *complementary*. The movement of life with the continual adaptation of internal to external relations in order to maintain homeostasis—that is evolution. This fusion of past and present principles then begs the question: is there any form of true Osteopathy that isn't, by nature, 'classical'?

~

With an understanding of the word, we can now examine one of the most primary osteopathic principles, that of the self-protecting and self-regulating mechanisms of the body (Kuchera, 2). From his fourth and final published work, *Osteopathy, Research and Practice* (1910), Dr. Still alludes to this concept:

> Osteopathy is to me a very sacred science. It is sacred because it is a healing power through all nature. (7)

Similarly, in his second publication, *Philosophy of Osteopathy* (1899), he speaks of his realization that the body itself is the fundamental healer:

> But at last I took my stand on this rock and my confidence in nature. (13)

Here, Still describes his turn to nature as he nears the end of his pursuit of wellness through the medicine of his time. Instead, he pursues his osteopathic approach to healing.

A belief in anything requires that believers plant their feet and stand firm—the only question being where to plant one's feet. Osteopathy, in the words of Dr. Still, is rooted in the bedrock of natural law. This is, in essence, the primary principle of osteopathic treatment: the body has the entrenched ability to self-heal and self-regulate of its own accord.

How does such self-regulation occur?

> The Osteopath has his own symptomatology. He seeks the cause, removes the obstruction, and lets Nature's remedy—arterial blood—be the doctor. (*Osteopathy, Research and Practice*, 5)

Any manual treatment has a physical, neuromuscular, and (although perhaps speculative) psychological change resulting in a nuanced physiological change that invokes an entire body response. Dr. Still says that the remedial life-giving force that exists within the body, invoked by that physiological change, is delivered by blood. Therein lies the approach to osteopathic treatment: if the self-healing and self-regulating mechanism of the body (which Still argues is facilitated by the blood) is being obstructed, then it is the job of the Osteopath to remove manually the obstructions or occlusions that are preventing that mechanism from taking place.

Where, then, does this task of treatment for the Osteopath begin? To answer this question we can look to the words of Still.

> To find health should be the object of the doctor. Anyone can find disease. (*Philosophy of Osteopathy*, 17)

If it is not for *disease* that the operator is searching, then what is it that the operator seeks in order to treat a patient? First we should examine that word—disease—to fully comprehend Still's meaning. In layman's terms, a 'diseased' state is anything that is contrary to the state of 'ease'. Defined, 'ease' is:

The state of being comfortable as freedom from pain or discomfort, freedom from care, freedom from labor or difficulty, freedom from embarrassment or constraint, an easy fit. (*Merriam-Webster*, 2014)

Medically, 'disease' has a more rigorous definition:

> An impairment of the normal state of the living animal or plant body or one of its parts that interrupts or modifies the performance of the vital functions, is typically manifested by distinguishing signs and symptoms, and is a response to environmental factors (as malnutrition, industrial hazards, or climate), to specific infective agents (as worms, bacteria, or viruses), to inherent defects of the organism (as genetic anomalies), or combinations of these factors. (*Merriam-Webster Medical*, 2014)

The osteopathic perspective on *disease* is quite different; in fact, the osteopathic perspective focuses not on disease, but on *health*. Rather than looking for disease, Osteopathy involves revitalizing areas where health is obstructed. Osteopathy is not alone in this perspective. Many organizations that promote global health take a similar holistic approach. Indeed,

> The World Health Organization (WHO) defines health as a state of complete physical, mental, and social well-being and not merely the absence of disease or infirmity. (*Constitution of the World Health Organization*, 1)

This perspective on health, from an international body that is invested in the wellness of the entire globe, was documented nearly fifty years after Still's writings. Yet like the WHO, Still and classical Osteopathy do not associate merely the absence of disease as a state of health. Modern forms of healthcare have instead, essentially, become sciences of disease because they focus not on the vitality (or inherent health) of the patient, but on pathological signs and symptoms, which are then categorized so that a precedented treatment can be administered to alleviate those symptoms. Dr. Still describes the allopathic approach to healthcare in his day:

> He looks on, and treats winter diseases with powerful purgatives, sweats, blisters, hot and cold applications with a view to remove congesting fluids. He is not very certain which team of medical power he can depend on. He hitches up many kinds of drugs hoping that a few of them may be able to carry the burden. He bridles his horses with opium, loads them down with purgative powders, and whips them through with castor oil, and for fear they will not travel fast enough he uses as a spur a delicately formed instrument known as the hypodermic syringe. He punches and prods until his horses fall exhausted. Disease and death should give him a large pension for the assistance he has rendered in their service. All is guess work whose father and mother are 'Tradition and Ignorance'. Ignorance of the kind that is wholly inexcusable to anyone but a medical doctor. (*Philosophy of Osteopathy*, 71)

With this osteopathic understanding of health and disease, let's return to the original question posed: where does the task of treatment for the Osteopath begin?

Disease, osteopathically, is an obstruction to the inherent self-healing and self-regulating mechanisms of the body, mechanisms that are instilled by nature. The Osteopath finds such obstructions physically by looking for and diagnosing structural abnormalities through palpation; this is why it is essential that Osteopaths have a pristine understanding of anatomy so that they can recognize the normal from the abnormal. Obstructions, restrictions, or dysfunctions will affect the self-healing and self-regulating mechanisms of the body, resulting in weakened tissue that will in turn provide a breeding ground for disease. Through their sound understanding of functional anatomy and physiology, combined with a developed sense of palpation (which can only come from years of clinical experience), Osteopaths can objectively identify restrictions, and restore health to these areas mechanically, anatomically, and physiologically. The body can then function at its optimal capacity. In Still's words, the *doctor* should aim to reconstitute and revitalize the inherent health of patients—their self-healing and self-regulating mechanisms—by treating the cause rather than treating the symptoms, the latter of which merely relieves the effects of a compromised state. What better way to offer true relief than to remove the obstruction that is holding the body from achieving its optimal state of health?

Osteopathic thinking sees pathology and health as two sides of the same coin: pathology exists within the body that is trying (but struggling) to survive, whereas health exists within the body that is thriving at survival. This healthy body represents the difference between stability and instability, equilibrium and disequilibrium. A stable equilibrium means the healthy body has the ability to return to a balanced state after a disturbance; it has the capacity to adapt, smoothly and functionally, and to generate enough energy to respond appropriately to physical, mental, and spiritual stress. Osteopathy treats the patient's lesion with the understanding that when the host is strong, disease cannot take root.

Where other forms of healthcare use synthetics or adjuncts as a way of suppressing the symptoms, Osteopathy uses manual therapy to stimulate the inherent mechanisms of the body. Osteopathic treatment not only has the ability to 'put out the fire' in the body that is illness—which is where many other forms of modern healthcare also thrive—but can remediate, refurnish, maintain, and prevent one's environment from causing future states of illness. In essence, the Osteopath aims to restore health to the patient rather than just eliminate symptoms of disease.

~

Classical Osteopathy is the science of association in that it acknowledges, examines, and determines the effects of the lesion but treats the cause. It is holistic rather than reductionist, which means that no one part of the body is favoured over another. Other therapies that separate the body into *just* muscles, *just* joints, *just* viscera, or *just* nerves sometimes lack the effectiveness that accompanies this holistic perspective. The body works as a unit, not in isolation, so it must be treated as a unit with all parts considered. Furthermore, Osteopathy incorporates a customizable approach to treating a patient because it understands that no two lesions are the same; for that reason, no two treatments can be the same. Therefore, each patient receives a unique osteopathic treatment, founded on principles, that is appropriate for that patient's body.

Let's explore once again the writings of Dr. Still as he enumerates the nine platforms of Osteopathy:

First: We believe in sanitation and hygiene.

Second: We are opposed to the use of drugs as remedial agencies.

Third: We are opposed to vaccinations.

Fourth: We are opposed to the use of serums in the treatment of disease. Nature furnishes its own serums if we know how to deliver them.

Fifth: We realize that many cases require surgical treatment and therefore advocate it as a last resort. We believe many surgical operations are unnecessarily performed and that many operations can be avoided by osteopathic treatment.

Sixth: The Osteopath does not depend on electricity, X-radiance, hydrotherapy or other adjuncts, but relies on osteopathic measures in the treatment of disease.

Seventh: We have an amiable attitude toward other non-drug, natural methods of healing, but we do not incorporate any other methods into our system. We are all opposed to drugs; in that respect, at least, all natural, non-harmful methods occupy the same ground. The fundamental principles of Osteopathy are different from those of any other system and the cause of disease is considered from one standpoint: disease is the result of anatomical abnormalities followed by physiological discord. To cure disease the abnormal parts must be adjusted to the normal. Methods that are entirely different in principle have no place in the osteopathic system.

Eighth: Osteopathy is an independent system and can be applied to all conditions of disease, including purely surgical cases, and in these cases surgery is but a branch of Osteopathy.

Ninth: We believe that our therapeutic house is just large enough for Osteopathy; when other methods are brought in, that much Osteopathy must move out. (Revised from *Osteopathy, Research and Practice*, 13-20)

Before we explore the relevance of these platforms, the reader must understand that they were written in the context of medicine in Still's time; moreover, these platforms encapsulate the stance that Dr. Still felt he needed to take to reinforce osteopathic practice in his day. The infiltration of other *adjuncts* into the *house* of Osteopathy was at the forefront of the American School of Osteopathy as they became more profitable than Still's '10-fingered Osteopathy'. However profitable, these adjuncts went against the principles of osteopathic treatment and, for that reason, are outside the grounds of classical Osteopathy. One could posit that the pursuit of wellness today has become incorporated into the healthcare industry, meaning that there are numerous modalities, products, or appliances that are available to today's patients. As Still contends, any of these adjuncts that follow the *natural methods of healing*, natural law, and the structure-to-function relationship are within the realm of an osteopathic approach to healing.

If we consider Still's nine platforms of Osteopathy in conjunction with the notion that osteopathic treatment is unique for each patient, we can conclude that osteopathic thinking requires the recognition of cases in which other forms of intervention are appropriate and in the best interest of the patient. The thinking Osteopath must be reasonable, rational, and never let his or her personal philosophies obstruct treatment of the patient.

I saw the brain of a man of success on a dish and a great golden plate or banner floating to the breeze. At the top of the plate I saw a picture of a man's brain—not his brother's brain, nor his doctor's brain, nor his preacher's brain, nor the brain of a general, nor was it the brains of a rich uncle, but the brain of a man who had been used to success in all things, and the words of the inscription said: 'This is of no use to others, it is no better than others only in one way, he had the courage to use it and let all others alone'. (*Autobiography of A.T. Still*, 1897: 55)

There are cases in which it would cause more detriment to the patient to ignore other aspects of modern medicine; accordingly, osteopathic treatment can be a complementary therapy to help the patient attain the best outcome. In these instances, osteopathic thinking can be used to determine the mechanism by which the case—or the cause—presented itself and what we can do for that patient to prevent the illness and its effects from reoccurring.

The goal of the Osteopath should be to restore health to the patient by following the principles of natural law. The more success we achieve on this front, the more the classical osteopathic movement will be reinvigorated in a rational way so that Osteopathy is regarded as complementary healthcare rather than alternative healthcare. How different our society's approach to health would be if, one day, other healthcare practitioners embraced the same rationale with respect to complementary treatment. If we wish to have this frame of mind permeate all forms of healthcare, we must begin within the classical osteopathic movement, aligned under the common goal of using principles-based classical Osteopathy.

A Methodology for Correction

A Necessary Methodology

As outlined in the preamble, this handbook acts as a guide in the delivery of general treatment. Before delving into specifics, however, the reader should have a broad understanding of the principles governing the methodology of treatment. Having a methodology ensures that the operator is not interpreting the ailment erroneously, delivering a series of prescribed techniques, and making individual corrections in isolation. Instead, having a methodology ensures that the operator has a rational thought process and delivers the necessary treatment based on how—and, more importantly, the reasons *why*—the patient presents the problem. In order to progress through one or a series of successful treatments, a methodology based on logical mechanics, anatomy, and physiology is needed.

Assessment and Reassessment

First off, the importance of observation as a tool of treatment must be stressed. The first and last steps in osteopathic treatment is observation as a means to obtain a diagnosis or assessment. Essentially, the operator must have an understanding of the lesion, as well as the tools to reevaluate or reassess for post-treatment effectiveness, before treatment can be delivered successfully. Observation begins within the first interaction between the operator and the patient; this includes taking note of their stature and both verbal and non-verbal communication. In addition to their palpatory findings, these observations help the operator build a clinical picture of the patient.

Although observation is an important clinical tool, it is equally important that the operator not offer a diagnosis too quickly. Part of building a *clinical picture* is to assess the patient in varying positions to generate an overall blueprint of how the soft and hard tissues are contributing to the pattern. While there are some observations that are more relevant than others, everything that the operator observes adds to the lesion picture. It is the job of the operator to distinguish the contributions of more significance from those of lesser significance by working through a differential diagnosis. What this means is that a constant interplay between assessment, treatment, and reassessment is necessary.

Osteopathic treatment uses four main criteria when diagnosing a lesion: asymmetry, restriction in motion, tissue texture change, and sensorial changes (Kuchera, 19). These four criteria are indispensable for establishing an osteopathic lesion or diagnosing a somatic dysfunction, and must be considered part of the operator's honed understanding of functional anatomy, physiology, and clinical experience. Often the easiest application of these four criteria is to determine asymmetry in tissues that, once palpated, should be motion tested to assess for functional movement. Since we can logically associate functional movement with functional physiology, little to no motion in an area will mean a restriction in the anatomical structures, which will have a corresponding restriction in the physiological processes of the body. The tissue covering a lesioned area will often undergo a change in terms of its physical texture; consequently, the patient may experience altered subjective sensory or motor function to the area.

From this initial diagnosis, the operator can use the wide variety of tools available to deliver treatment in the most safe, effective, and efficient manner according to the particular case. This includes elements like positioning of the patient (whether supine, prone, sidelying, or seated) using a direct, indirect, or balanced approach based on whether it is an acute or chronic condition. Whether the patient should actively participate in the treatment or be passive will be assessed through the communication available between the operator and the patient. Nevertheless, the operator's choice of leverage is crucial; sometimes a short lever is the most effective means of creating an adjustment over a longer lever, or vice-versa. Regardless of which method operators choose to apply their treatment, they should have a rational thought process that is based on the diagnosis obtained from their initial observations and palpation appraisal.

Once treatment has been delivered the operator must again use the tools of observation and palpation, only this time to reevaluate and reassess in order to determine if the treatment was successful. This sequential movement through assessment, treatment, and reassessment is crucial to evaluate the effectiveness of treatment, and to see if the operator must choose a different treatment tool. It is important to note that assessment and treatment of an area can look, to an observer, much like the same thing; to the operator, however, assessment and treatment differ in their approaches to the barrier, and are just two of the technical skills the operator must master in terms of clinical experience.

Technical Application

An operator must be both technical and tactical in their delivery of effective treatment. In other words, in addition to their rational approach they must also have polished manual skills. Much like the rational methods, these manual skills are governed by principles, such as connecting the lever to the fulcrum, evaluating rhythm, and assessing the barrier.

When determining the use of leverage, the operator must acknowledge which lever, whether short or long, is more appropriate to deliver the intended treatment. Should the operator approach treatment with a long lever, it is necessary to first recognize whether the lever is functional before adjustment should be attempted. Additionally, generating leverage is only effective if the operator has an established (or fixed) point through which force will be applied, rather than simply generating leverage and having it disperse in different directions. Furthermore, using the lever system for adjustment must be done with a rhythm that puts the patient at ease. This principle not only addresses the pace by which the operator alternates between diagnosis and treatment, but also the way in which operators approach the barrier (whether in a position of ease or bind). Rhythm is one factor that determines the difference between *imposing* treatment or having the patient *accept* the treatment.

Another component of the operator's technical ability involves treatment dosage. As with any form of medicine, knowing how much or how little, in addition to how often the operator provides treatment, is a skill acquired over the course of one's practice. Generally, acute cases often require a weaker, shorter, and more indirect approach than chronic cases, the latter of which the operator applies a longer, more direct treatment less frequently. Although these are general guidelines for dosage, there are no set rules in treatment. Dosage depends on the patient's lesion, constitution, and vitality, as well as the technical ability of the operator.

Developing a honed sense of palpation is also a technical skill. There is a significant difference in sensory reception depending on whether the operator intends to deliver a stimulatory touch (light and repetitive pressure) or an inhibitory touch (slow, deep, sustained pressure). It is imperative that the operator chooses the correct form of palpation in order to generate the intended response.

Over time, and with much practice and clinical experience, these principles of technical application will become more refined. Developing these manual skills is critical for evaluating whether the patient's health improves as a result of technical application on the operator's part, the operator's approach to the lesion pattern, or the patient's own constitution and vitality. With sound manual skills, operators can rely on their technical ability and thus change their tactical approach to better deliver effective treatment.

Staging

Staging refers to the patient's position during treatment. Staging (which includes supine, prone, sidelying, and seated positions) is yet another important aspect of methodology; however, each comes with its advantages and disadvantages when applied to different tissues. Each position should have an objective—and thus, a rationale—behind why that position is being utilized.

Supine position (Chapter Three) provides the operator with an opportunity to work on the flexion stage of the lesion, as extension is limited by the position of the table on the dorsal aspect of the patient. As gravity travels through the body from anterior to posterior, it places the spine in a flexed position, bringing load off of the facets and onto the soft tissue on the dorsal aspect of the spine (**FIG 1.1**). In this position, then, supine can be used to address the soft tissue that holds the hard tissue using flexion, sidebending, and rotation in the sagittal, coronal, and transverse planes respectively. An example of this occurs during a supine leg rotation (page 44); we use the legs as levers to manipulate the pelvis and the lumbar spine, often oscillating the leg in different planes to affect each joint within its primary motion. The primary motion corresponds directly to the structure of the articulating surfaces, so by using leverage in the same plane as the primary motion we

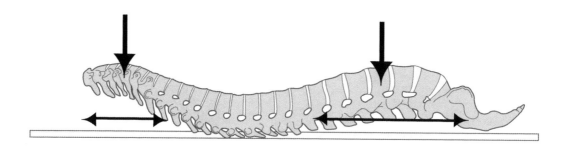

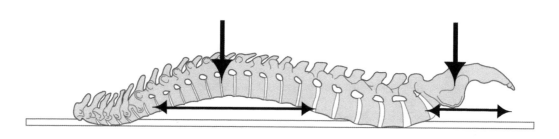

FIG 1.1: *Positioning using gravitational force in supine (top) and prone (bottom) position.* Since gravity travels differently through the body in each of these positions, the operator can stage them over the course of treatment

can conjointly address the soft and hard tissues of the area. The soft tissue restriction, if present, will be reached prior to the hard tissue restriction because of the anatomical relationship of the two tissues in the supine position (the soft being posterior to the hard), as gravity travels from anterior to posterior through the body.

On the contrary, prone position (Chapter Four) allows us to not only have a better visual of, and physical contact with, the spine, but also places it in an extended position as gravity travels from posterior to anterior through the body. In a similar but contrary fashion (as explained in supine position), gravity places the load back onto the facets as the table acts as an abutment to flexion; as such, prone position can be used to address the spine—especially after the larger, soft tissues have been addressed in supine position—this time using extension in the sagittal plane, along with sidebending and rotation. Prone allows the operator to focus particularly on the hard tissue lesions and the more intrinsic soft tissues such as the intrinsic musculature, ligaments, and joint capsules, any of which may be holding those hard tissue lesions.

Lateral and seated position (not shown in this handbook) are advantageous because the table does not abut movement in any plane, be it flexion, extension, sidebending, or rotation. This means that operators can address the soft or hard tissues concurrently. Often, lateral and seated positions are used to coordinate the soft and hard tissues of the spine once either of those tissues have been addressed separately in the preceding positions.

The operator should have an idea of the advantages and disadvantages of each position so that he or she can choose which one will deliver effective treatment. This staging of positions sequentially, over the course of one or several treatments, relies on the operator's understanding of the role of mechanics, anatomy, and physiology as it relates to the patient's lesion pattern.

Mechanics, Anatomy, and Physiology

An osteopathic treatment calls for the operator to possess a mind similar to that of a tradesman, be it mechanic, plumber, electrician, and so on. The operator must examine the way forces travel through, and interact with, an area of the body and to what degree they influence the neurovascular structures that supply and extract nourishment to and from those areas. In other words, a mechanical lesion will generate a physiological response, producing signs and symptoms that indicate where operators should focus their efforts. The symptom provides the clue as to what is taking place physiologically, yet we use our palpation of the anatomy to assess for the best approach, and then apply technical skills (mechanics) to deliver the necessary treatment.

This process can be regarded as a triad made up of mechanics, anatomy, and physiology, all of which become a schematic for treatment. Oftentimes, patients will present a combination of signs and symptoms, which are the result of obstructed physiology due to some anatomical interference that stems from a mechanical occlusion. This is known as *mechanopathology*—where a mechanical disturbance causes an impaired physiological effect—and explains how mechanics become one of the major factors in directing the course of treatment through anatomical justification and physiological reasoning. Mechanopathology is another tool through which the operator determines differential diagnoses; as they assess, deliver their treatment, and reassess, operators can determine whether their mechanical, anatomical, and physiological reasoning was effective, or if they must explore an alternative route.

This means of differential diagnosis also helps operators determine if they have identified a *cause* or an *effect* of the lesion. In palliative cases, working on the effects of the lesion may be an ideal route, but if the operator would instead like to make structural changes, then he or she must address not the effect of the lesion, but why the lesion is there. Treating the *effects* as a list of independent *causes* will not always be as effective as pinpointing the cause in which the effects are rooted.

Changing this way of approaching the lesion will help operators to correlate the lesions and thus change their delivery of treatment; if the operator continues to treat an area and observes no change, then the lesion is likely being propagated from somewhere else. This is a progression that relies on pristine technical abilities on the operator's part, for if operators know that they have applied their treatment correctly, yet they have not been successful in producing a change, they can move on and keep searching for the cause of the lesion.

The mechanics, anatomy, and physiology must be correlated to one another in the three-dimensional structure of the human body. First, the mechanics: *what is loading the area?* Second, the anatomy: *what anatomical discord is present as a result of the mechanical influence?* Finally, the physiology: *what effect is the anatomical discord having on the neural or vascular control of the respective area?* All of these aspects are rooted in mechanics, as they can all continue to perpetuate a mechanical imbalance.

Correlation and Coordination

We must keep at the front of our mind the practice of correlating individual structures within the overall superstructure of the human body. Since structures with more mass tend to have a larger mechanical influence on the overall superstructure than the smaller structures, it would be pertinent to focus our attention primarily on these larger structures if we wish to make a significant mechanical change. Through the lens of this logic, we can concentrate our attention on the pelvis as the foundation of our general treatment. From this focal point we can work from cephalad to caudad, and from the axial skeleton to the periphery, otherwise known as the *base-up, centre-out* principle.

The pelvis, being the innominates with respect to the sacral keystone, has an influence on both the upper and lower body. Consequently, it plays a notable role in the distribution of force between these two areas. It stabilizes our legs during the walking cycle, carrying the weight of one leg while apportioning the load of the spine, thorax, upper limbs, and cranium to the other. Because of its substantial mechanical influence on the body, the pelvis (or lower T-line) should be the basis of constitutional treatment in order to have the largest mechanical effect on a patient's anatomy.

From a biomechanical point of view, the pelvis has the most influence on the superstructure of the human body; from a neurovascular point of view, the spine is a passageway from the control centre to the periphery for the delivery of information that will dictate physiological functions. In order for the spine to carry out its role, it must be treated as a centre of coordination rather than a centre of correction, meaning that it should be tuned as a collection of articulations that, when functioning optimally, will allow the correct physiological functions to occur.

This principle explains why the pelvic adjustment is the basis for treatment and why, after the pelvic adjustment, we work through the spine to affect the periphery. From the pelvic adjustment we can integrate the lumbar adjustment to influence the coordination of movement in the lower limbs. Coordination is further facilitated by the neurological mechanisms passing through the lumbosacral plexus. Building upon a solid lumbopelvic adjustment, the operator can then work upwards to the thoracic adjustment, and build up to the upper T-line to stimulate the parietal and visceral fields of the region (neurologically through the autonomic nervous system, and mechanically through the osseous rib cage). Once we reach the cervical spine, we are again affecting the coordination of movement to the limbs through the neurology—this time, the upper limbs through the brachial plexus—in addition to having prepared the thorax for the drainage that will be necessary in the succeeding cervical and cranial adjustment. Adjustment involves the law of balancing each part of the body with equal importance. No one part is privileged over another.

Drainage and Supply

This direction of treatment is also crucial from the perspective of drainage and supply of the one active and two passive fluids in the body: arterial, venous, and lymphatic, respectively. Fluid will flow in the path of least resistance, and thus a pathway free of obstruction is necessary in order for 'old' fluid to drain and create space into which 'new' fluid can flow to supply the area. Working on passive circulation is a means of addressing active circulation. As Still states:

> The rule of the artery is absolute, universal, and it must be unobstructed or disease will result. I proclaimed then and there that all nerves depended wholly on the arterial system for their qualities, such as sensation, nutrition, and motion, even though by the law of reciprocity they furnished force, nutrition, and sensation to the artery itself.
> (*Autobiography of Andrew Taylor Still*, 1908: 182)

Allowing for fresh blood to reach the tissues is a means of restoring health to areas of dysfunction. For this reason, treatment should progress in a way that addresses drainage of distal areas preceding direct treatment of those areas.

Sequencing, Phasing, and Spiral Thinking

This way of working through the body and utilizing the tools of technical application is known as sequencing. Sequencing allows operators to be sequentially specific in their delivery of treatment. Similarly, phasing—the ordering of treatment over a series of treatments—allows operators to tailor their treatment specifically to each patient over time.

Both of these aspects of treatment utilize a spiral thinking pattern referred to as *global, local,* and *focal.* Operators must configure the treatment so that they can observe different characteristics of the lesion; this multidimensional view will help to decipher how each component interacts with the overall lesion pattern. For example, globally the operator can address larger structures, such as the orientation of the upper and lower T-lines and how they display from a general perspective. Locally, they can examine the curves of the spine and their relation to one another, i.e., through comparing or contrasting the anterior or posterior curves and how they may or may not be compensating for one another. Focally, the operator can move into intersegmental assessment or examination of the peripheral joints.

This method of thinking is essential, as the operator must be able to oscillate between general and specific assessments and treatments in order to learn whether certain structures are the *cause* or the *result* of other mechanical, anatomical, or physiological discord within the body. Often we must look at long lines of myofascial tissue and clear any asymmetries or restrictions in this global pattern before we move on to the orientation of the more focal, intrinsic soft tissues (for example, muscular or ligamentous, or even osseous hard tissues). We follow this procedure because their *focal* asymmetry may be a product of a more *global* asymmetry. Co-ordination of the upper and lower girdles and the spinal curves should be addressed before the vertical line can be attended. This mode of thinking is only possible if the operator has the ability to spiral in and out, to treat any aspect of the body with all of the available tools, using global, local, and focal thinking.

At this point the reader should recognize that this methodology for constitutional treatment is dictated not only via the mechanics of combining and distributing forces, but also through the anatomical approach of addressing the soft and hard tissues (which will be further explained in the *Myogon Model,* page 26). The reader should also appreciate the interplay of physiological principles—in this case, the neurology—that are based upon Still's dictums of structure influencing function. By addressing the spine, the operator has affected the environment housing the neurological input and output that controls the distal structures. This is another instance where adjustment to the distal structures must start from the central structure where the operator can have the greatest impact, sometimes with the least amount of treatment.

Stabilization

One aspect of osteopathic treatment that makes the practice unique from other forms of manual therapy is the concept of stabilization. Stability concerns the ability of a body, when disturbed from a state of equilibrium, to revert back to (restore) its original condition. This concept of restoration is similar to practices of homeostasis, wherein cells and tissues adapt to live in harmony and balance—a function that is as true for one cell as it is for the entire organism.

The methodology put forth in this handbook is based in and around the operator's ability to effect small, consistent changes to the body that will result in a stable structure—a structure that, when stimulated to a point outside of its stable environment, is able to return to balance easily. Stabilization means that the body can withstand whatever comes its way: stability equals resilience. It should be the aim of the operator to guide patients, through treatment, into a position where it is difficult for them to become *destabilized*.

If the body truly does work as a unit (Kuchera, 2), then the body should be treated as one entity, with all its parts considered within the context of the whole. There is no one part of the body that can be worked on in isolation, as the entire lesion pattern must be addressed. Using global, local, and focal thinking requires correlational treatment of individual structures in an effort to stabilize the entire structure. Instead of only treating individual effects in a local or focal environment using techniques, areas of dysfunction must be considered symbiotically within the global structure in order to provide a treatment that leads to stabilization.

It is also important to remember that osteopathic treatment is an *evolution* rather than a *revolution*; osteopathic treatments are not always immediately adjustive, but instead eventually lead to stabilization. The osteopathic treatment does not take place when the patient is on the table, but rather through somatic (bodily) responses after the treatment is applied. For this reason, the patient must be given enough time to respond to treatment (sometimes on the scale of hours to days) in order for the physiological changes from the treatment to stabilize. Applying more treatment before these changes have occurred may not always result in stabilization, and for that reason the frequency of treatment is crucial. Remember that the body is the self-healing and self-regulating mechanism; the operator is simply the facilitator.

A Rational Methodology

It should now be evident that a rational methodology is necessary in delivering an effective osteopathic treatment. Again, in the words of Dr. Still, reconstituting the circulation must be the primary objective of the Osteopath, as it is the vital life force through which the Osteopath can assist the body in restoring health:

> He seeks the cause, removes the obstruction, and lets Nature's remedy—arterial blood—be the doctor. (*Osteopathy, Research and Practice*, 5)

By addressing the body through a general treatment methodology that takes into consideration any mechanical or neural compressions on the circulation, the operator can encourage the movement of arterial blood to restore the body's constitution and vitality. This approach allows the operator to use a wide variety of tools rather than techniques, and fosters a malleable thought process where operators can respond to findings rather than execute a predetermined routine. The operator must always have a plan regarding their course of treatment, and a rationale for why they are taking that course. For this reason, treatment begins with methodology.

General Treatment: An Introduction

General treatment is an important part of osteopathic history and heritage. It provides the practitioner with a basis for practice, can be used to improve the constitution and vitality of the patient, and integrates (and correlates) the entire structure. General treatment has multiple implications from both a therapeutic and diagnostic perspective. As we will explore, classical osteopathic literature and general treatment, in keeping with Dr. Still's philosophy, could even be referenced as 'general diagnosis'.

General Treatment In Classical Osteopathic Literature

One point that should be made first is that there is little to no reference, in any of the classical osteopathic literature, to Dr. Still doing anything resembling a 'general treatment' (or anything with similar terminology). It may seem contradictory, then, that this text, being osteopathic in nature, is attempting to extrapolate such a term while subscribing to Stillian principles. We will explore Still's writings, specifically *Osteopathy, Research and Practice* (1910), to gain an understanding of his approach and how it can be connected to general treatment. For now, we can consider that

> It is of unlimited importance that you search every joint from the atlas to the coccyx and know that every vertebra is in its proper place, every rib in perfect articulation. (255)

In this particular excerpt, Still is referring to his approach in treating conditions of the lungs. His choice of the word *search* is of utmost importance; it implies that he *looks* for the *perfect articulation*—that being the movement between tissue surfaces—in each and every joint of the body. However, this does not necessarily mean that he *treats* each and every joint in the body. Instead, he *explores* or diagnoses every joint, every tissue, and all of their articulations, but only *treats* or adjusts as needed. There are far more instances than merely treatment of the lungs where Still uses this approach. Consider the excerpts below.

In the case of consumption:

> Now I will say no more to the skilled osteopath than to tell him to begin with his work on the consumptive patient at the neck, and *explore*[1] and *adjust* the atlas and all joints of the spine and ribs from the head to the coccyx. (299)

---

[1] Italics have been added to these excerpts in an effort to draw the reader's attention to particular diction or phrases of immediate relevance. The italics do not appear in the original text.

In instances of constipation:

> In treating constipation I began with the atlas because *I could find somewhere between the occiput and the coccyx,* obstructive causes that would prohibit the production and the delivery of the unnatural lubricating fluids to the large and small intestines. (362)

For typhus fever:

> I continue the *exploration* and *adjustment* all along the neck and entire extent of the spine from the sacrum and coccyx. (872)

In diseases of the sweat glands:

> When a patient comes to me suffering from a perverted condition of the sweat glandular system, without hesitation I proceed to *examine the whole spinal system* of bones beginning with the coccyx. ... After leaving the coccyx I am just as careful to seek and obtain perfect adjustment of the innominate and sacrum. After this I take up the lumbar and adjust every section of that region. Then I most carefully *explore* and *adjust* every vertebra from there on up the spine to the atlas. (490)

With the treatment of women in stages of menopause:

> With these facts before us we must *explore* and *adjust* all articulations beginning with the head and atlas, and continuing to all joints of the neck, spine and ribs clear through the lumbar to the sacrum and coccyx. (515)

For patients with neurasthenia:

> In all cases of hysteria, sick headache, and all other conditions along the line of this whole list of nerve disturbances I find much variation from a truly normal spine *beginning my work with the coccyx and ending it with the atlas.* (627)

And rheumatism:

> I *examine* every bone and every joint from the occiput to the coccyx. (658)

Dr. Still recounts these and other cases—such as dysentery (370), hemorrhoids (532), and so on—where he employs these methods of examining the entire body. From these excerpts the reader can derive two main points of Still's osteopathic treatment.

First: no matter the condition the patient presents, or the area in which there seems to be the largest disturbance, Dr. Still explores all regions of the body for lesioning. Whether the condition originates from the cranium, the thorax, the pelvis, or other locations, he leaves no area of the body unexamined.

Second: although he *explores* each and every articulation, he only *adjusts* that which needs adjusting rather than treating the entire body. Here we can identify Still's rational approach. General treatment can be regarded as general diagnosis, a way in which to explore the lesion pattern of the entire body, whereby the operator uses this diagnosis to treat that which needs to be treated. If we use general treatment as a way of treating anything and everything in the body, we have diverged from the foundation of osteopathic thinking. Conversely, if we take this principle as the foundation for our general treatment, we are remaining true to osteopathic, Stillian philosophy.

Regardless of the absence of the term 'general treatment' in the literature, there were times in which Dr. Still did use a general approach. Ultimately, there were occasions when he treated more *generally* and occasions when he treated more *specifically*. In any case, the phraseology is not what should distract us from searching for a Stillian approach to treatment, for he did not employ the terms *general* or *specific* with respect to treatment. Still delivered *osteopathic* treatment. We can ascertain from his writing that what he wanted the student and practitioner to avoid was fragmentation: taking pieces of treatment and applying them to different parts of the body with no rhyme or reason. He wanted the operator never to be frivolous or haphazard, but instead to minimize invasiveness while generating the most positive effect.

In keeping with the classical literature, this means that classical Osteopaths need to make sure that everything they do, even with general treatment, has a cause and a reason. Osteopathic practitioners are not simply going through the motions of a specified *routine*, but instead are reflecting on why they are doing what they are doing, and what information or goal they intend to gain from doing so.

Instances Calling for General Treatment

Reading further into classical osteopathic literature, Carl McConnell and Charles Teall—two of the earliest Osteopaths who were thus influenced by Dr. Still—discuss their take on what general treatment entails, and the cases in which it should be delivered to the patient. In their book, *The Practice of Osteopathy* (1906), they write:

> The only explanation of such a procedure that one can think of is a lack of conception as to what osteopathy really is. To give a general treatment in every case is not only actually detrimental to the patient but it is the height of folly on the osteopath's part, for it gets him into a slovenly habit of procedure from both scientific and curative points of view, besides giving the outside world an impression that osteopathy is but little different from massage and Swedish movements instead of skillful, mechanical engineering of the human body.

> A general treatment, broadly speaking, should be given only under three conditions: (1) Constitutional diseases that are to be treated symptomatically. (2) Anemic cases. (3) When one is ignorant of the real cause of the disease. Each of these conditions is self-evident why a general treatment should be given. A fourth might be added, for those individuals who think they are not getting value received unless they are treated from head to foot. Such patients are usually ignorant of the philosophy of osteopathy and it is the osteopath's duty to teach them differently.

> The general treatment consists in stretching the spinal column from the

atlas to the coccyx and relaxing all contracted muscles along both sides of the spinal column, besides giving special treatment to the cervical region, between the scapulae, the splanchnics and internal and external rotation of the legs. It is no wonder that fake osteopaths do cure a case occasionally. They are quite certain to correct some disorder by pulling and hauling a patient around in such a manner. (69)

McConnell and Teall strongly advocate that general treatment, dispensed within a practice that fraudulently refers to itself as Osteopathy, reveals the folly of the practitioner rather than the practice of true, classical Osteopathy. To administer a general treatment in *every* treatment for *every* patient disregards instances when a specific rather than general approach is necessary. Instead of solely performing general treatment, McConnell and Teall suggest three or four primary occasions wherein general treatment is appropriate.

First, general treatment can be used to build up the constitution and vitality of a patient overall. By going through the body in a collective but sequential way, the treatment can stir circulation and improve nourishment to and from all tissues, thus improving overall health. In the cases of anemia, improved circulation will help to enhance the delivery of nutrients to tissues that may be compromised by the existing condition. The operator works in this general manner in an effort to remove enough lesioning and dysfunction to mobilize the body's natural ability to self-heal and self-correct—in essence, to restore the patient's constitution and vitality.

On the other hand, general treatment can also be used as a tool to palliate. In instances where a patient possesses a fairly weak constitution and vitality, sometimes doing specific treatment very locally (or focally) can become too overwhelming and result in destabilization. In these cases, general or constitutional treatment is the safest, most effective, and most efficient tool for that patient, and the objective of treatment is to provide the patient with more days of better quality.

General treatment, moreover, has as much of a role to play in diagnostics as it does in treatment. Often, practitioners will rush to judgment in order to identify the lesion so that they can immediately apply the appropriate treatment. In some ways, this mode of thought strays from osteopathic thinking. If we regard the body as a self-healing and self-regulating mechanism, and if we provide treatment that allows it to function better collectively, then these lesions for which we have specific diagnoses (the minutia) will be taken care of as well. Often a patient will display a variety of lesions that are the result of a pre-existing lesion. These associated lesions only clutter and make it more difficult to decipher the overall lesion pattern. For the purposes of diagnosis, general treatment has its most optimal effect when we are trying to reduce clutter, for it is ideal for practitioners to clear the smoke in order to have something firm upon which to base their work. Perhaps general treatment should be redefined from something practitioners perform when they cannot provide a correct diagnosis, to something they offer when a diagnosis is not practical to make. General treatment, then, is not for times when the practitioner is unsure of the treatment, but is for times when the practitioner has chosen general treatment in order to clear the clutter and make a correct diagnosis.

With respect to diagnosis, general treatment has additional efficacy, particularly in the earliest stages of treatment. Upon initial contact with the patient, the operator has limited foresight in terms of how the patient will respond to treatment. There are, of course, general guidelines that the practitioner can follow to dispense the dosage of treatment, so to speak. Guidelines to consider might include whether the patient exhibits an acute or chronic condition; thus, how they might react to treatment will be more difficult to determine in the initial stages of the procedure. For this reason, operators should use general treatment as a starting point on which they can base the course of the succeeding treatments after the patient's body has an opportunity to respond. It is important that if the practitioner utilizes general treatment in such cases, he or she should not resort back to a general approach more than is necessary as a means to deliver treatment thereafter.

As practitioners in today's mechanized world, we have to keep in mind that we are working with people of different constitutions than those with whom Still was working. People of Still's day were much stronger and robust owing to lifestyles that involved heavier labour when compared to today. In true osteopathic fashion, we need to evolve our thinking with our context (the lifestyles of whichever society we live in). We must evolve to treat the people of today, who may or may not have less robust constitutions than those in Dr. Still's day. Because of this evolution, there is no better time in our history to apply general treatment, otherwise known as *constitutional treatment*, to build up the body's structural framework and integrity. The entire idea of general treatment is to improve overall mobility and circulation, to encourage the body to function at a higher level collectively, and to regard the body as a holistic structure with interdependent physiology.

Application of General Treatment

General treatment need not be lengthy, but can be administered regularly, especially in the earlier stages of treatment. As with any treatment, it should be relaxing to the patient so that the practitioner does not fight the lesion and mistakenly become fixated on one area of the body. One of the benefits of general treatment is that it illustrates the full story of the lesion pattern by addressing all aspects of the body. When practitioners work in this general fashion they can address the limbs and examine how, for example, they oppose the axial skeleton, or how the limbs and the axial skeleton work collectively. This can help the practitioner understand, on the table, the lesion mechanics within the entire lesion pattern. In other words, operators can look not just at the pelvic lesion, but at how that lesion might be affecting the limbs, the cranium, or even the viscera.

In order for us to use the limbs, it must be ensured that the levers are, in fact, an effective tool for diagnosing the axial skeleton. Although 'general treatment' is usually synonymous with 'the entire body', we can still isolate procedures as a general lower limb treatment, a general upper limb treatment, a general cervical treatment, a general cranial treatment, etc. All of these approaches are viable options, but for the thinking Osteopath a general treatment provides a basis from which to begin treatment globally, then locally, and then (if required) globally again. General (global) treatment can provide a methodology by which we can diagnose and treat all areas of the body, but we must have an overall picture of where to focus in, when to zoom out, and, more importantly, where to go next.

This is how we can refer to general treatment as being *sequentially specific*, meaning that the operator correlates structure and function throughout the entire body. For example, the operator may adjust the pelvis specifically, but must then adjust the pelvis to the lumbar spine, the lumbar spine to the thoracic spine and shoulder girdle, the cervical spine to the thoracic spine, and so on. Treatment now takes on a progressive, logical, flowing thought process: it is sequentially specific.

A Unique General Treatment

It is important to understand that the *modus operandi* behind general treatment provided in this handbook should not be confused with the idea of general treatment as a *routine*. We can maintain a methodology without general treatment becoming predetermined and, accordingly, deliver a unique treatment tailored to each patient. Within the context of this principle, we can utilize global, local, and focal thinking to make specific treatments within that general treatment. In the same way that we would use a different magnification on a microscope to look at the same specimen, we use these different lenses to shift our way of thinking about the lesion pattern. If we can analyze the lesion pattern from these different perspectives, then no general treatment should look the same for each patient. Therefore, the treatment should exercise differing means of integration, correlation, and coordination each and every time; each general treatment, although non-specific, adopts a different approach. In order to devise a methodology with these gradations of focus, we need the ability to increase and decrease optical intensity (figuratively speaking). It is only then that we will build a better understanding of the lesion in a mechanical, anatomical, and physiological context.

Myogon Model

An important concept pertaining to the methodology behind general treatment from a mechanical, anatomical, and physiological perspective is found within the Myogon Model. The Myogon Model was developed by Robert Johnston through his study of Classical Osteopathy, his readings of Still, his interactions with John Wernham and the theory of compensation, his clinical experience, and his grounded understanding of functional anatomy.

From his clinical experience, Mr. Johnston found that patients with hip dysfunctions invariably show signs of dysfunction in the opposing shoulder (and vice versa). A torsional line exists within these patients, extending from one hip to the opposite shoulder, from which it can be deduced that the body moves through planes and axes of a long diagonal torsion. The Myogon Model provides a functional anatomical explanation for why these cases with correlating lesions present themselves with such persistence.

The myogons themselves are polygons, or triangular structures, that exist within the muscular framework of the body. Myogons are affiliated with the structure-to-function relationship of shapes and mechanics, where triangles provide structural support and stability; essentially, they describe the relationships of anatomical structures and mechanical lines. The myogons provide a rational methodology for working through the body. These polygons, one triangle inverted on top of another, are made up of soft tissue lateral lines that bind together the hard tissue structures from the upper girdle to the lower girdle (**FIG 1.2**).

The lower myogon is represented by the lines of force that follow quadratus lumborum and the iliopsoas, while the upper myogon is represented by trapezius and pectoralis major (anterior and posterior respectively). These muscles connect the upper T-line, which extends across the acromion processes of one shoulder to the other, and the lower T-line, which extends from one femoral head to the other. Although we can name specific musculature that may contribute more than others to these myogons, it is important to remember that, functionally, these triangles represent lines of force from groups of muscles rather than one muscle working in isolation. Similarly, although we can name specific hard tissue structures that comprise the upper and lower T-lines, these specific bony landmarks are used as a tool to place emphasis on any distortion in the asymmetry from one side of the body to the other, particularly in the shoulder and pelvic girdle. These myogons, represented by both soft and hard tissue, intersect at the thoracolumbar junction, which acts as a pivot point through which these myogons have motion. With this in mind, we can draw lines of force that course through the body from one hip to the opposite shoulder.

In addition to these lateral lines, there are two vertical lines (one anterior and one posterior) whose positioning is a direct result of the tension through the lines of pull already described. Anteriorly, this vertical line is represented by soft and hard tissue that extends from the chin—through to the sternum, the linea alba, and the pubic bone—while posteriorly the vertical line is represented by the soft and hard tissues of the spine. Distortions of the aforementioned lateral lines in any direction will have a direct influence on the position of these vertical lines, anteriorly and posteriorly.

The idea of geometric shapes existing within the planes and axes of the body is not a novel concept. John Wernham referenced a system of polygons that existed in the coronal plane to describe vertebrae that act as pivots and keystones to balance the arches of the spine (Parsons, 2006). Furthermore, the idea of recurrent patterns of dysfunction occurring in the body is a concept well established by Dr. Gordon Zink in his discussions of the Common Compensatory Pattern (Zink, 1979). These concepts are related directly to the precursory writings of Dr. Still:

> Does man have in him some kind of chemical laboratory that can turn out such products as he needs to fill all his physical demands? If by heat, exercise, or any other cause he gets warm, can that chemistry cool him to normal? If too cold, can it warm him? Can it adjust him to heat?
> (*Philosophy of Osteopathy*, 85)

Dr. Still sees the body as a biological compensatory structure that adjusts to the internal and external environment as required—a fundamental component of a self-healing and self-regulating mechanism. In its optimal state the body should, ideally, be able to revert back from any extreme to a point of balance. In cases of dysfunction, he speaks of the body's inability to revert and the necessity of manual treatment to restore heat to cold areas. This is one example of a compensatory situation:

> As I began at the bases of the brain, and thought by pressures and rubbings I could push some of the hot to the cold places, and in doing so I found rigid and loose places on the muscles and ligaments of the whole spine, while the lumbar was in a very congested condition. (*Autobiography of A.T. Still*, 1897: 51)

During the development of the Myogon Model, rather than study the writings of Wernham, Zink, and Dr. Still in isolation, Mr. Johnston focused on the common principle that linked all of these models: compensation.

Compensation is the coupling of equal and opposite resultants in the body: hot and cold, mobility and stability, flexed and extended, sidebent and rotated, compressed and in tension. Even more than that, the capacity of a body to compensate is represented by its ability to adapt to stimuli while not hindering its ability to adapt to future stresses. Nearly everyone has some sort of dysfunction or lesion pattern for which their body must compensate on a daily basis; many of us are 'functionally dysfunctional'. A body that is not compensating well for these dysfunctions may allow stimuli of a lesser magnitude, which otherwise would be able to adapt, to express themselves somatically, but only because the entire structure is already compromised. On the other hand, a body that is compensating is persistently able to adapt to its environment. Much of our ability to compensate relies on our constitution and vitality in relation to how well we adapt to stimuli, and how dysfunctions express themselves.

As the operator works through the body using the myogon lines represented by the anatomy, they are truthfully working on patterns of compensation. For example, where there is tension on one lateral line, there should be compression on the equal and opposite lateral line in the body. If these lines are unequal there will be disharmony in the entire structure. This disharmony often leads to chronic and erratic states of fluctuation indicative of a non-compensatory lesion pattern. In these cases, it becomes the work of the operator to bring those lines back into balance in order for the treatment to have a therapeutic effect.

The Myogon Model was developed in an effort to reduce the amount of labour involved in treatment, to give the operator direction for a better diagnosis (and a better palpation), and facilitate a better delivery of treatment. It provides the operator with a method of differential diagnosis, for if the operator has a sequence by which to gauge the physiology rather than giving a full body adjustment or general treatment every time, he or she can better determine the effectiveness of the treatment.

The following chapters will discuss general treatment using the aforementioned methodology and application of this Myogon Model as a direction for the delivery of osteopathic treatment.

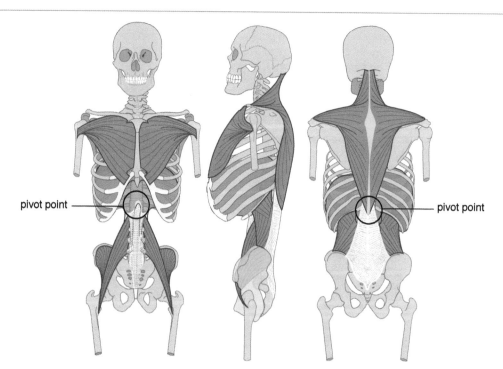

pivot point

pivot point

FIG 1.2: *Myogons from an anterior, posterior, and coronal perspective.* Anteriorly, the upper and lower lateral lines are made of the pectorals and iliopsoas, respectively *(left)*. Posteriorly, the upper and lower lateral lines are made up of the trapezius and quadratus lumborum, respectively *(right)*. The intersection of these two polygons, commonly referred to as the confluence of force, lies at the thoracolumbar junction and the diaphragm *(centre)*.

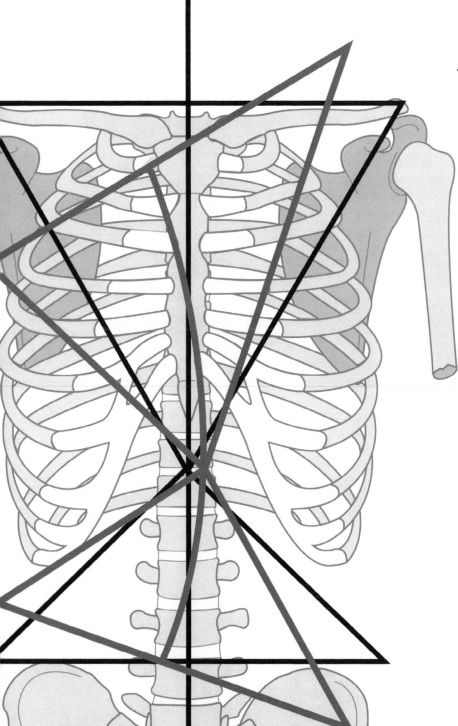

Initial Intake

The initial contact between the operator and the patient is vitally important. It must be colloquial, not clinical, and the operator should display the utmost respect to the patient through gestures such as using the patient's surname, shaking hands, and making direct eye contact (**FIG 2.1**). All of these subtleties are of great importance for the practitioner, as valuable information about the patient can be gleaned before even beginning a formal 'intake'.

A formal medical history is of value to the case, but the practitioner should still aim to maintain as colloquial a disposition as possible; this will set the tone for open dialogue with the patient. The medical history can be perused, but the discussion they have with the patient (to assess their constitution and vitality) is of greater value. The trophicity of their tissues, the tone of their voice, and their body language can be interpreted not unlike the written intake. Even before the practitioner begins their formal Osteopathic Structural Diagnosis, the initial intake with the patient is the start of diagnosis.

The practitioner should also have a discussion outlining what he[1] will be trying to achieve for the patient. Practitioners should be able to answer any queries the patient may have— questions as simply as *'What is Osteopathy?'*—in order to make the patient more comfortable, and to elucidate the goals they are aiming to achieve over the course of treatment. The practitioner should explain to the patient his objective of facilitating the self-healing and self-regulating capacity of her own body.

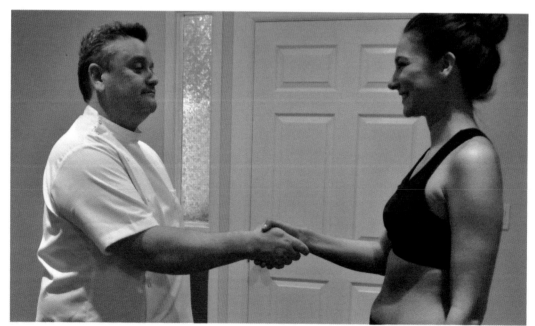

FIG 2.1: *Initial Intake.*

[1] Because the operator depicted in this handbook is male, the gendered pronouns 'he/his/him' have been used to maintain grammatical integrity between antecedents and pronouns. The same pronoun gendering occurs with respect to the female patient depicted.

Initial Test for Red Flags

Before operators begin their patient/passive assessment, they should gain an understanding of how the patients can move of their own accord. To do this, the operator can have the patient perform a series of motions as a form of patient-active assessment. Oftentimes, many of these tests are performed on the initial consultation, or after a series of treatments, as a form of initial assessment when practitioners first meet the patient, or to evaluate the effectiveness of the operator's treatment.

Before any motion tests are performed, the operator can have patients shift weight to their toes such that they are plantarflexing their ankles, and then drop back on their heels (**FIG 2.2**). If the patient exhibits any pain, especially in the abdominal or lower back region, it can indicate a dysfunction that may accompany a disc herniation, nerve compression, or even an abnormal growth. Many of these notably serious conditions will exhibit a sharp, localized pain upon the patient dropping onto her heels. The operator should adjust his course of treatment according to the findings.

Next, the operator will have the patient perform a series of global motion tests to assess the patient's overall mobility. It should be noted that in several cases, many patients will not be able to perform some of these motions, so the operator should adjust the course of treatment accordingly.

First, the patient squats as far as is comfortable toward the floor (**FIG 2.3**). This assesses global flexion of nearly all the joints in the body, from dorsiflexion of the ankle, to flexion up the lower limb into the pelvis, upper limb, neck, and head. After this, the patient stands and goes into a position of extension in all of the joints of their body to similarly assess global extension (**FIG 2.4**).

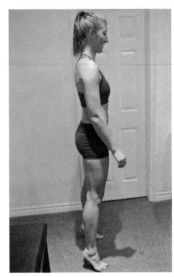

FIG 2.2: *Heel drop.*

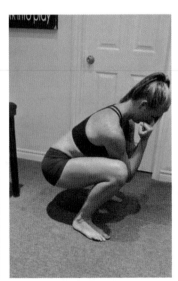

FIG 2.3: *Global evaluation of flexion.*

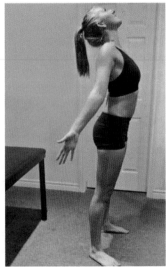

FIG 2.4: *Global evaluation of extension.*

The operator can unilaterally assess the motion in all planes of the lower and upper limbs by having patients balance on one leg while they flex their knee and externally rotate their hip, and then perform a 'backstroke' with their arms (**FIG 2.5, 2.6**). Lastly, the operator can have the patient flex, extend, sidebend, and rotate her head to assess motion of the neck (**FIG 2.7**).

During all of these movements, the operator should take note of any restrictions or asymmetries patients may exhibit as a global assessment of their range of motion, for it will be necessary to amend and assess their treatment and progress accordingly.

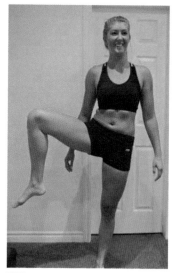 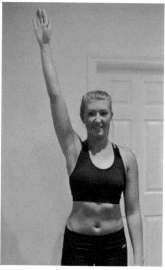 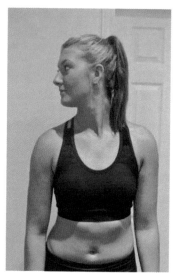

FIG 2.5   **FIG 2.6**   **FIG 2.7**

Patient active dynamic evaluation of lower extremity (left), upper extremity (centre), head, and neck (right).

Patient Set-Up

The way in which the patient is set up on the table (whether in supine, prone, sidelying, seated, or even during a standing evaluation) is important for the diagnosis and delivery of treatment. Thus, a short time must be taken to set the patient in the correct position. Patient set-up should not be regarded as a *routine,* but as a means of putting the patient into position so that the operator can exercise control during the treatment.

During a standing evaluation the operator should have the patient stand as far away as necessary to acquire a global understanding of how gravity affects the patient while upright. When the patient moves onto the table for a seated evaluation, the operator should again be far enough back to see how the patient now *sits* in gravity. The patients' initial position of how they present themselves can be used as a point of assessment, as they will sit, stand, or lie comfortably in the posture of their choosing (some patients will splay a limb asymmetrically from one side to another, some will exhibit global sidebending or rotation, and so on). The operator can use this observation as diagnostic tools for patients' lesions, as they will position themselves in a manner that accommodates their lesion pattern most comfortably.

Once the operator is ready for the next phase, the patient should be set up in a position that is as close to neutral as possible so that treatment can be delivered from a neutral starting point. The operator should adjust the patient to neutral with respect to the position of their limbs, hips, shoulders, and spine—but of course 'neutral' will vary from patient to patient. Pillows can be used to provide patient comfort or to normalize the spine; in supine, for example, the pillow should be placed under the occiput, whereas in prone it is often placed under the lumbar spine. In both cases, the pillows are used to bring the spine out of flexion or extension and into neutral.

Although time should be allotted for patient set-up, operators should be efficient so that they can move swiftly into the next step of their treatment.

Standing Evaluation

We obtain an understanding of patients and their response to treatment by our evaluations pre- and post-treatment. Therefore, it is often said that osteopathic treatment begins and ends with observation. When the practitioner is observing the patient in a standing position, it is important that the patient presents herself in a way that she feels comfortable so that the operator can properly assess the T-lines. This means the operator may need to evaluate the patient through layers of clothing as efficiently as possible, for the more time the operator takes to evaluate, or the less clothes a patient is wearing, the more chance there is to react to the operator's observations, and thus, to alter the patient's stature. The operator should make an effort to take a mental image of the patient's T-lines (consider them and their contribution to the overall lesion pattern), and then move on.

Static: T-Lines

The T-lines themselves consist of two horizontal lines, one stretching across the acromion processes in the upper girdle, and the other across the iliac crests in the lower girdle; and two vertical lines, one extending from the patient's chin to their pubic bone on the anterior, and the other to their spine on the posterior (**FIG 2.8, 2.9**). These lines tell us how horizontal and vertical (respectively) the body is in space. In other words, they indicate how torque and tension lines are interacting with the framework of the body under gravity.

Within these T-lines we are looking for deviations from each of these planes (**FIG 2.10**). This means that in the horizontal plane we are looking for declinations while in the vertical plane we are looking for flexions and extensions (rotation and sidebending), both unilaterally and bilaterally. In theory, if the patient's T-lines are oriented within these two planes with no dysfunction present, the structures designed to carry the load are functioning as intended. In reality, however, any deviation from these planes will cause a shift in the load-bearing within the framework of the body. A declination off of the horizontal line, for example, will indicate a shift in the vertical line; this structure, particularly under strain, is not intended

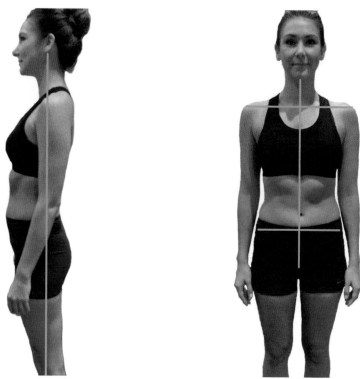

FIG 2.8   **FIG 2.9**

Static assessment of the vertical upper and lower T-lines (left), horizontal T-lines (right).

to carry that type of load.

It is important to recognize that any declination of the horizontal line or shift in the vertical line will load differently on the joints of the periphery (such as the hip, knee, and ankle). Consequently, including these peripheral joints with the T-lines in the overall assessment is beneficial. Very often in treatment, the primary adjustment is meant to coordinate the upper and lower girdles with one another before the secondary adjustment to the peripheral lines takes place. Situations where this approach may not be sufficient occur when there is a pre-existing dysfunction in the periphery, such as a trauma to the knee, that then causes a shift in the T-lines up the chain. This is known as an ascending lesion versus a descending lesion, whereby a dysfunction in the pelvis would cause a shift in weight-bearing on the knee. In these instances it may be beneficial to work from the periphery inwards, but even then, in cases where acute traumas become chronic, we often have to return to adjusting the T-lines and work from the centre outwards. Working from the centre outwards is necessary because there is a greater influence transmitted from the pelvis to the knee than there is from the knee to the pelvis. This concept originates from the principle that, in the physical world, structures with a larger mass have a greater influence on the overall superstructure than those with a smaller mass. This is true for the human body as well; the magnitude of the effect from the pelvis is greater than the magnitude of the effect from the knee joint. Thus, treatment begins with establishing elasticity and plasticity at this larger structure.

By superimposing these lines—which are, in essence, mechanical lines of pull or force—over the top of the body, the practitioner can use these T-lines as a blueprint from which to base and assess the progress of treatment. If we can bring these lines back into position, the myofascial tension within this blueprint can be alleviated, and often many of the local or focal deviations in the hard structure will be either clearer to the practitioner or alleviated altogether.

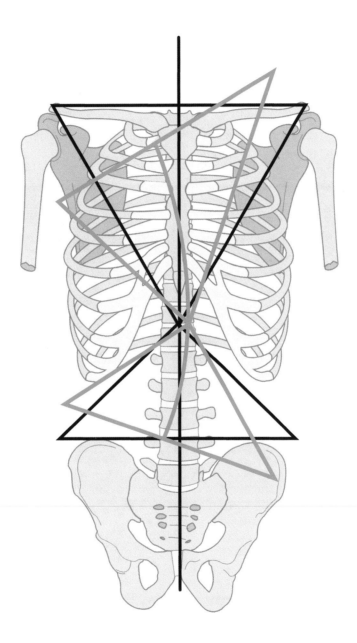

FIG 2.10: *Deviations of the horizontal and vertical lines.* The green lines indicate how a declination in the upper and lower T-lines can cause a deviation in the vertical line or T-lines, indicated in black. These declinations shift the load to other structures and cause an imbalance in the lines of force.

Dynamic: Motion Testing

Operators can also incorporate an active-dynamic evaluation of the T-lines. With their hands in a flank hold over the innominates, operators can stabilize the pelvis and have the patient, whose arms are crossed, rotate in each direction on a vertical axis (**FIG 2.11, 2.12**). By doing this, we can assess the upper T-line in relation to the lower T-line. We can also assess the rotation itself for the quality of one side when compared to the other. This approach is founded on the principles of diagnosing a lesion, which includes assessment of asymmetry and restriction in motion.

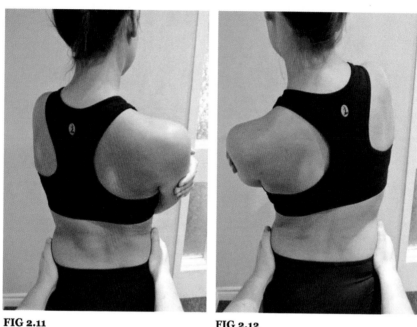

FIG 2.11   **FIG 2.12**

Patient active-dynamic of motion testing of the T-lines in a standing position.

Keeping in mind the normal physiological motion in the thoracolumbar region, rotation to one side is coupled with sidebending to the opposite side (**FIG 2.13**). This means that the distance on the side to which the patient is rotating, or the convexity, is longer from the acromion to the iliac crest than the distance between those same points on the opposite side (the side of the sidebending or concavity). For the sake of efficiency, the operator needs only to use one plane of motion to gather information in multiple planes.

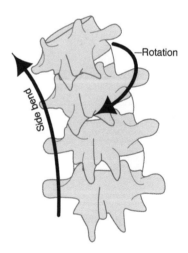

FIG 2.13: *Motion mechanics of the thoracolumbar region.* Sidebending and rotation are coupled to opposite sides in the thoracolumbar region in the absence of extreme flexion or extension due to the structure and orientation of the articulating facets.

Seated Evaluation

The seated evaluation, both statically and dynamically, follows the same principles as the standing evaluation, but now the operator can assess the T-lines as the patient straddles the table. Now that the patient is essentially sitting on her pelvis rather than standing on her feet, changes in the pattern of the T-lines can be noted. If the pattern has changed from what the operator observed in the standing evaluation, we can surmise that a dysfunction in the legs is making a larger contribution to the overall lesion pattern. The position of the patient is also important for the dynamic motion test, wherein the operator has the patient, like in the standing evaluation, turn from one side to the other. This straddle position locks the two innominates in place on the table so that the innominates themselves, as well as the legs, have little to no motion when the rest of the spine moves. For this reason, a seated position gives us a *true spinal* evaluation, whereas in a standing position the involvement of the legs does not necessarily give us the truest spinal diagnosis. This helps the operator to differentiate whether the lesion is being generated from the spine, the pelvis, or the legs—an observation that will assist the delivery of treatment.

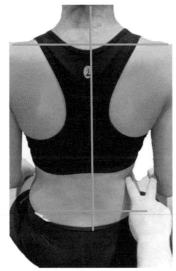

FIG 2.14: *Static assessment of the T-lines in a seated position.*

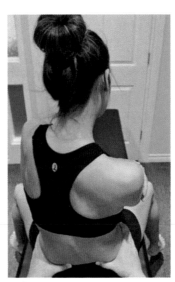

FIG 2.15

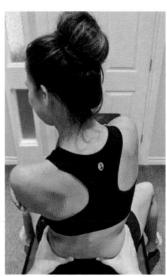

FIG 2.16

Patient active dynamic motion testing of the T-lines in a seated position.

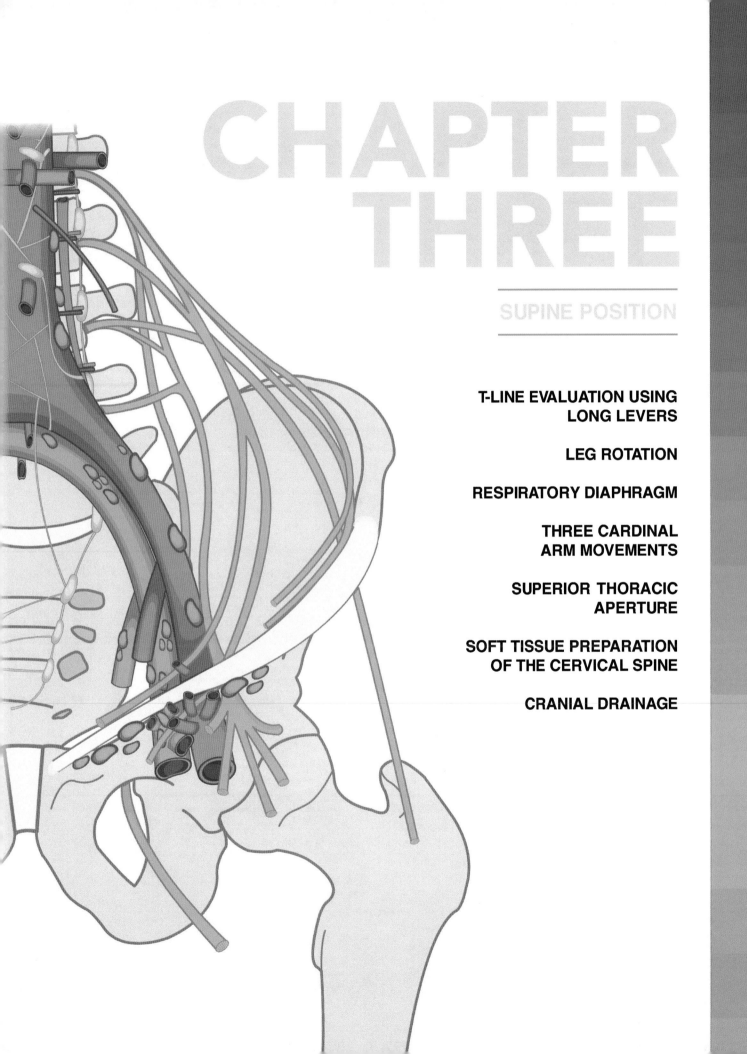

CHAPTER THREE

SUPINE POSITION

T-Line Evaluation Using Long Levers

The following images illustrate the evaluation of upper and lower T-lines using long levers with the patient in supine position.

Lower T-Line

The operator can use the patient's legs to generally assess the position of the lower T-line for asymmetries or restriction in motion.

Cupping with a light hold and straight arms at the calcaneus, the operator uses his body to produce a lean-back pressure that tractions through the patient to the baseline. It is imperative that the operator leans back with his entire body rather than exerting muscular strength during this assessment (**FIG 3.1, 3.2**). Operators can do this maneuver unilaterally or bilaterally as a form of long chain diagnostics, assessing from the foot to the coxofemoral joint—and even up into the lumbar spine—all from the end of the table. Bilaterally, the operator can compare the two sides, particularly how the traction travels up the chain simultaneously.

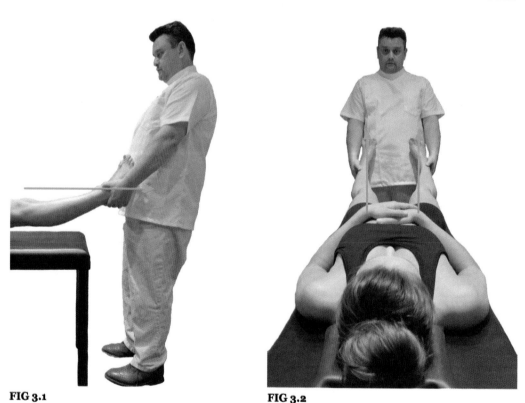

FIG 3.1   **FIG 3.2**

Using lean-back pressure to assess the lower T-line bilaterally using long levers in supine position.

Unilaterally, operators must change their hand position to better isolate the movement to one side at a time (**FIG 3.3**). With one hand on the calcaneus, the other on the talus, and arms tight to the body, the operator can place the patient's other leg on his own ASIS. As the operator rotates with his body, he can create a tractional force through the position of the leg in his hands while blocking movement at the patient's other leg. This motion can be compared to that of a telescope: when pulled at its end, all of the lenses follow within their designated range, which results in an elongation of the telescope (**FIG 3.4**). The connections of these lenses that create the telescope can be thought of as the joints in the leg that create a chain. A functional leg will have gapping, or elasticity, through all of the joints in the chain (talar, tibiofemoral, coxofemoral, lumbar, etc.), wherein a loss in elasticity signifies some type of lesion along that chain.

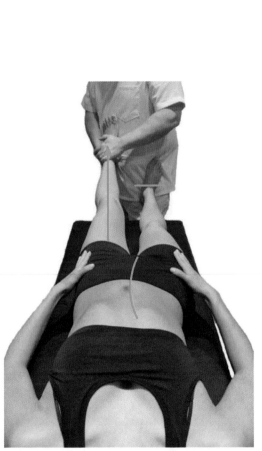

FIG 3.3: *Telescoping unilaterally in a caudad direction to assess the lower T-line using a long lever in supine position.* The operator uses traction to create right sidebending.

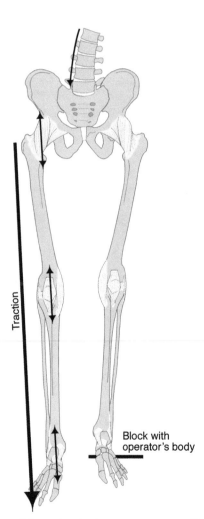

Traction

Block with operator's body

FIG 3.4: *Telescoping.* As the operator rotates with his body, he creates a tractional force through the leg in his hands while abutting movement at the patient's other leg.

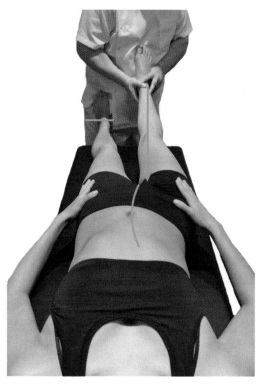

FIG 3.5: *Telescoping unilaterally in a cephalad direction to the lower T-line using a long lever in supine position.* The operator uses cephalad pressure to create the right sidebending position.

Just as easily as the operator creates traction in a caudad direction, he can also turn toward the patient and create a force, through the patient, in a cephalad direction. This technique assesses the pliability of the structures within the chain as they are compressed (**FIG 3.5**).

Aside from telescoping, the operator can also use the legs to assess the long lever by arching them from the patient's midline. Holding both legs by the calcaneus in an *A-frame stance*, in which the feet are shoulder-width apart and weight is distributed evenly between both feet, the operator creates traction through the legs with lean-back pressure, and then deviates the legs to either side (**FIG 3.6, 3.7, 3.8**). The side to which the operator deviates creates traction down the opposite side of the table (i.e., moving to the operator's right creates traction down the patient's right leg). Owing to this traction, the operator can assess the long lateral line, or tension in the coronal plane, down that side.

Whether the operator assesses unilaterally or bilaterally using the legs, if they are to identify an asymmetry or restriction in motion, the operator might suspect that there is a lesion somewhere in the chain of the lower limb, and a corresponding resultant in the lower T-line. Should the operator use enough force, he will be able to influence the lumbar spine and assess for flexion or extension (if using the lower limbs bilaterally) or sidebending and rotation (if using them unilaterally).

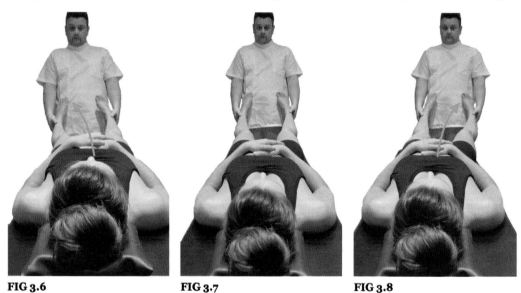

FIG 3.6   **FIG 3.7**   **FIG 3.8**

Arching to bilaterally assess the lower T-line using long levers in supine position. The operator moves from neutral *(centre)* to either side *(left, right)* to assess tension on the lateral lines.

Upper T-Line

Similar to using the lower limbs to assess the lower T-line, the operator can use the patient's upper limbs to assess the position of the upper T-line (**FIG 3.9**). In this case, the operator cups with a light hold and straight arms at the carpals, and uses lean-back pressure to telescope the right and left arms and down the lateral lines.

Depending on the patient's assessment, one arm may not 'telescope'. This would indicate (just as it did with the legs) a lesion in the chain on that side. To further investigate where this lesioning originates, we can use the compensation theory and the Myogon Model; by using the oblique lines and vertical lines to connect the two horizontal lines, the operator would be led from one shoulder through the central pivot to the opposite hip to investigate the source of lesioning (**FIG 3.10**).

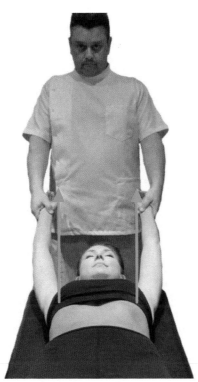

FIG 3.9: *Using lean-back pressure to assess the upper T-line bilaterally using long levers in supine position.*

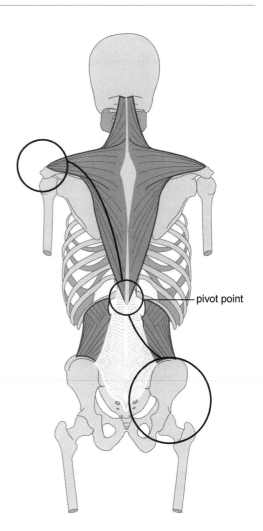

pivot point

FIG 3.10: *Applying the Myogon Model.* In this example, if the operator found lesioning in the patient's left shoulder he may wish to investigate the right hip because of the muscular connections and lines of force that connect these two points.

Leg Rotation

During a leg rotation, the operator can use the leg as a long lever to assess and treat any joint up the chain. The operator can begin at the coxofemoral joint, the sacroiliac joint, the lumbosacral junction, or any of the joints of the lumbar spine.

Assessment begins as the operator picks up the patient's leg. Grasping on the inside of the ankle to cup the calcaneus, the operator is lateral to the table with straight arms and straight body lines in an A-frame stance (**FIG 3.11**). Through this stance, he can preliminarily assess the weight of the leg and restrictions in any plane of motion. The operator then turns uptable by pivoting on his inside leg. During this pivot he can also place his uptable hand delicately beneath the patient's popliteal fossa, all the while being mindful of body mechanics, and keeping himself oriented in straight lines (**FIG 3.12, 3.13**).

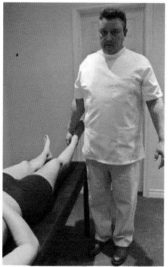 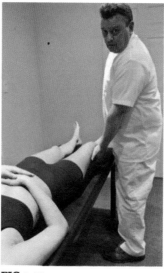 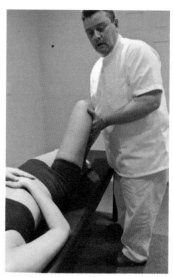

FIG 3.11: *Assessing the lower limb.*

FIG 3.12

Exercising control when picking up the leg.

FIG 3.13

The operator now needs to bring the leg into flexion at the knee such that the patient's foot is resting flat on the table. To do this, operators use their uptable hand, which they have placed in the popliteal fossa to buckle the leg at the knee, and will guide with both hands the leg into a flexed position as they take a step uptable. The operator should now be in an A-frame stance, facing squarely across the table with full control of the patient's leg (**FIG 3.14**).

The operator must now establish a fixed point. Standing with the patient's leg tight to their body, and while facing across the table, operators will use their downtable hand to clasp the knee and push the leg away across the table (**FIG 3.15**). This rocks the pelvis and lumbar spine into rotation, allowing operators to slide their uptable hand underneath the pelvis, sacrum, or lumbar spine to create a fixed point wherever they wish to direct their treatment.

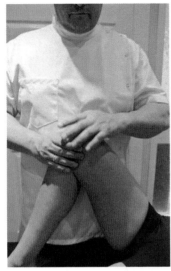

FIG 3.14: *Securing the patient's leg in an A-frame stance.*

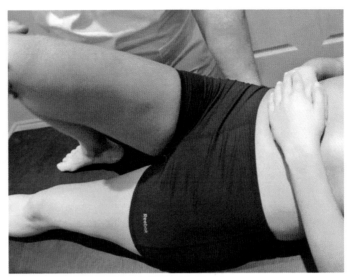

FIG 3.15: *Establishing the fixed point.*

With their fixed point established, the operator then rolls the pelvis and spine back onto the fixed point by bringing the leg back into the sagittal plane (**FIG 3.16**). At this juncture, operators must have the correct body mechanics, including a fencer stance with straight legs, and their body and uptable foot pointed in the direction of their intended corrective force. Cradling the knee, the operator pushes up and rests the patient's leg just below the tibial plateau in his own delto-pectoral groove. It is crucial that the operator does not rest the leg farther down than the tibial tuberosity. This is done to avoid hyper-flexion of the knee, especially in cases where there is already an existing trauma or dysfunction at that joint. The operator can use his opposite hand to reach across and stabilize the opposite ASIS, and to isolate the rocking to their intended location at the fixed point. The operator is now ready to assess and deliver the treatment.

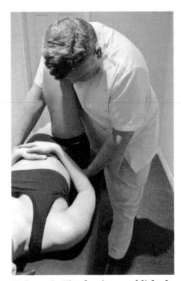

FIG 3.16: *Fixed point established with control of the lever*

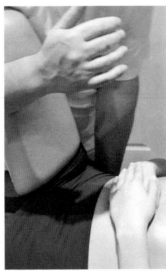

FIG 3.17

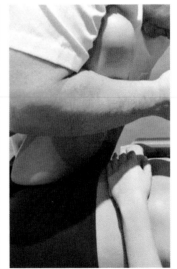

FIG 3.18

Bringing the leg into flexion to build tension in the sagittal plane.

Using his body to bring the hip into flexion in the sagittal plane, the operator feels to assess how far into this motion the patient can move until the barrier is reached (**FIG 3.17, 3.18**). After they have reached the barrier the operator can begin treatment through oscillation; using an on and off procedure, operators should adjust intensity to the tool of treatment deemed appropriate, be it a direct, an indirect, or a balanced approach.

The motion of the leg during a leg rotation varies in different areas of the pelvis and lumbar spine because rotation must correlate to the motion capabilities possessed in that area. For example, the coxofemoral joint is capable of motion in all three planes; the sacroiliac joint moves along the axes of the sacrum; the lumbosacral junction is more rotational; the mid-arch of the lumbar spine exhibits motion mostly in the sagittal plane; and the thoracolumbar junction has, again, more of a rotational dynamic (**FIG 3.19**). As such, oscillatory movement during a leg rotation should vary depending on the area to which the operator has directed a fixed point.

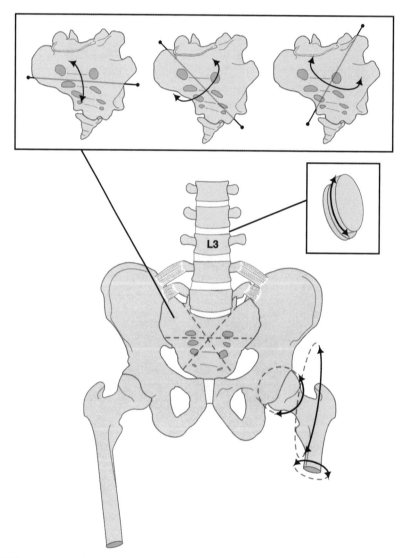

FIG 3.19: *Differences in motion capabilities in different areas of the pelvis and lumbar spine.* The oscillation of the leg rotation must coordinate to the motion capability of the joint at the fixed point.

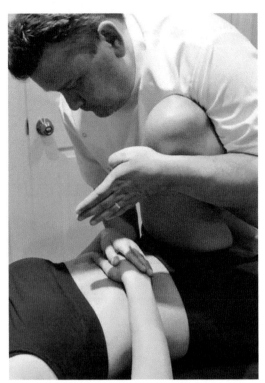

FIG 3.20: *Bringing the leg over midline, left side.*

It is important that operators, while creating an adjustment, maintain their position into or out of the barrier while being cognizant of the comfort and safety of the patient. It is crucial that operators establish the fixed point before they begin their oscillation, for they will use the barrier at that fixed point as a reference to compare progress after treatment has been delivered. If there has been a change to the barrier from the preliminary palpation before treatment, then the operator knows the treatment has been successful.

There are some considerations that the operator needs to appreciate when working on the left side of the patient versus the right. For example, when the patient's left leg is brought into flexion, it is important to bring the knee much farther over midline than was done with the right; this is to challenge the left—commonly more fibrosed—sacroiliac joint (**FIG 3.20**). Here, the operator can stop and hold to create myofascial tension that will warm, soften, and release the fibrotic tissues along the dorsal ligaments of the joint before heading back into the leg rotation. Whether operators rotate the femoral head in a clockwise or counterclockwise direction within the acetabulum is not of significant consequence, so long as they are using the leverage correctly to target the lesion according to their diagnosis.

It is also important when addressing the joints beyond the coxofemoral joint that there is sufficient tension loaded on the coxofemoral ligaments in order to elongate the lever enough to bring tension to joints past the hip (**FIG 3.21**). If there is not enough tension in the coxofemoral ligaments, there will never be enough leverage transferring through the leg and innominate to adjust the innominate, the sacrum, the lumbar spine, and so on. By nature of the anatomical orientation of the ligaments of the coxofemoral joint, often the operator must initiate internal rotation within the coxofemoral joint to channel the tension from the femoral head to the acetabulum. Keep in mind, however, that the direction to which the operator winds the ligament will vary from patient to patient. In some cases, the operator may not be able to establish sufficient tension on these ligaments because they have gained so much laxity, and have thus lost their stability due to the patient's diminished constitution or vitality. In these situations, short leverage as opposed to long leverage may be a better treatment tool for that patient.

Depending on how the operator would like to utilize the leg as a lever in correcting a dysfunction, he must be aware of the muscular tissues that are on and off tension during each stage of the leg rotation. Direct approaches to a lesion may require more tension on a muscle group to generate a line of force, for example, whereas indirect approaches may require a muscle group to be off tension (**FIG 3.22**).

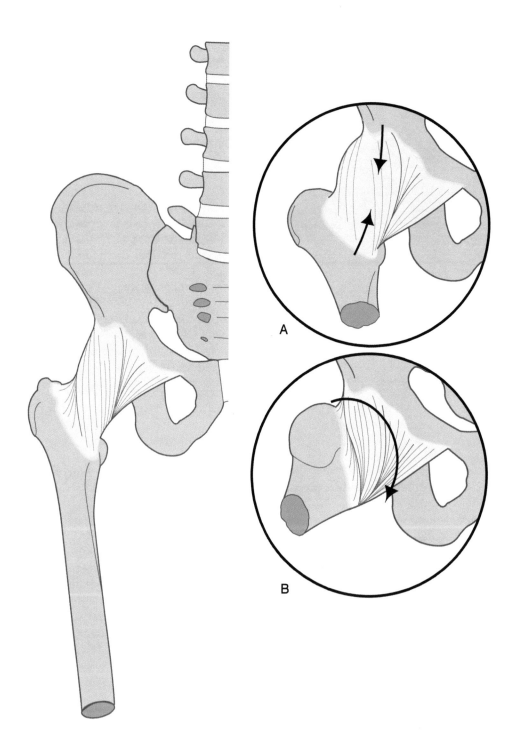

FIG 3.21: *Ligaments of the coxofemoral joint.* As the hip joint is brought into flexion, the surrounding ligaments are slackened as their attachment points are approximated (a). Often during a leg rotation the operator will need to induce internal rotation of the hip joint in order to build enough tension on these ligaments such that the force is transmitted from the leg through the joint and into the innominate (b).

Anatomy of the Leg Rotation: Musculature

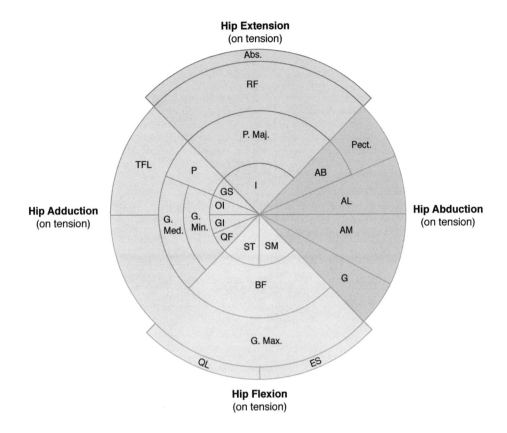

Hip Abduction			
Muscle	**Origin**	**Insertion**	**Innervation**
Pectineus	Pectineal line of the pubis	Pectineal line of the femur	Femoral and obturator (L2-L4)
Adductor Brevis	Body and inferior ramus of pubis	Pectineal line and proximal third of linea aspera	Obturator (L2-L4)
Adductor Longus	Body of pubis, inferior to pubic crest	Middle third of linea aspera	
Adductor Magnus	Inferior ramus of pubis, ischial ramus, and ischial tuberosity	Gluteal tuberosity, linea aspera, supracondylar line, and adductor tubercle	Obturator (L2-L4) and sciatic (L4-S3)
Gracilis	Body and inferior ramus of pubis	Tibial pes anserinus insertion (medially)	Obturator (L2-L4)

FIG 3.22 (a)

Hip Extension

Muscle	Origin	Insertion	Innervation
Abdominals	**External Oblique:** External surfaces ribs 5-12	**External Oblique:** Linea alba, rectus sheath, pubic tubercle, and iliac crest	**External Oblique:** Lower intercostal, iliohypogastric, and inguinal nerves
	Rectus Abdominis: Costal cartilages 5-7 and xiphoid process	**Rectus Abdominis:** Pubic tubercle	**Rectus Abdominis:** T5-T12 spinal nerves
	Internal Oblique: Thoracolumbar fascia, iliac crest, and inguinal ligament	**Internal Oblique:** Ribs 10-12, linea alba, rectus sheath, and the pubic tubercle	T7-L1 spinal nerves, iliohypogastric and ilioinguinal nerves (T12-L1)
	Transverse Abdominis: Thoracolumbar fascia, iliac crest, ribs 7-12, ASIS, and the inguinal ligament	**Transverse Abdominis:** Linea alba and pubic tubercle	
Rectus Femoris	AIIS and notch below	Base of the tibial tuberosity via patellar tendon	Femoral (L2-L4)
Psoas Major	Transverse processes, bodies, and intervertebral discs of lumbar vertebrae	Lesser trochanter	Femoral (L2-L4) and lumbar spinal nerves
Iliacus	Iliac crest and fossa	Lesser trochanter	

Hip Adduction

Muscle	Origin	Insertion	Innervation
Tensor Fasciae Latae	ASIS and iliac crest	IT band (lateral condyle of the tibia)	Superior Gluteal (L4-S1)
Gluteus Maximus	Iliac crest, dorsal surface of the sacrum and coccyx, and sacrotuberous ligament	IT band (lateral condyle of the tibia) and gluteal tuberosity	Inferior gluteal (L5-S2)
Gluteus Medius	External surface of the ilium, superiorly	Greater trochanter	Superior Gluteal (L4-S1)
Gluteus Minimus	External surface of the ilium, inferiorly	Greater trochanter	
Piriformis	Anterior surface of the sacrum	Greater trochanter	Nerve to piriformis (S1-S2)
Gemellus Superior	Ischial spine	Intertrochanteric fossa	Nerve to obturator internus (L5-S2)
Obturator Internus	Internal surface of obturator foramen and membrane	Greater trochanter	
Gemellus Inferior	Ischial tuberosity	Intertrochanteric fossa	Nerve to quadratus femoris (L4-S1)
Quadratus Femoris	Ischial tuberosity	Quadrate tubercle and intertrochanteric crest	

FIG 3.22 (b)

Hip Flexion			
Muscle	**Origin**	**Insertion**	**Innervation**
Erector Spinae	**Iliocostalis (lumborum, thoracis, and cervicis):** Sacrum, thoracolumbar fascia, and iliac crest	**Iliocostalis (lumborum, thoracis, and cervicis):** Angles of all ribs and TPs of C4-C7	Dorsal rami of the spinal nerves from the surrounding segments
	Longissimus (thoracis, cervicis, and capitis): Sacrum, thoracolumbar fascia, SPs of lumbar vertebrae, TPs of thoracic vertebrae, and articular pillars of C4-C7 vertebrae	**Longissimus (thoracis, cervicis, and capitis):** TPs of the lumbar vertebrae, 2-12 ribs between the tubercles and angles, the transverse processes of the cervical vertebrae, and the mastoid process of the occiput	
	Spinalis (thoracis and cervicis): SPs of T10-L3, T1-T2, and C5-C7	**Spinalis (thoracis and cervicis):** SPs of T2-T8 and C2-C5, spanning all vertebrae on the lateral aspect	
Quadratus Lumborum	Transverse process of lumbar vertebrae and 12th rib	Iliac crest	T12-L2 spinal nerves
Gluteus Maximus	Iliac crest, dorsal surface of the sacrum and coccyx, and sacrotuberous ligament	IT band (lateral condyle of the tibia) and gluteal tuberosity	Inferior gluteal (L5-S2)
Biceps Femoris	Ischial tuberosity (long head) and distal linea aspera (short head)	Fibular head	Sciatic (L4-S3) and common peroneal (L4-S2)
Semitendinosus	Ischial tuberosity	Tibial pes anserinus insertion (posteriorly)	Sciatic (L4-S3)
Semi-membranosus	Ischial tuberosity	Medial condyle of the tibia	

FIG 3.22 (c)

Anatomy of the Leg Rotation: Flexion Considerations of Ventral Structures

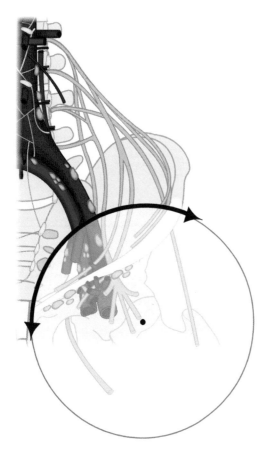

Considerations of structures placed under compression at the inguinal fold during flexion of the leg.

Iliohypogastric Nerve (L1)
Ilioinguinal Nerve (L1)
Genitofemoral Nerve (L1, L2)
Lateral Femoral Cutaneous Nerve (L2, L3)
Femoral Nerve (L2-L4)
Femoral Artery + branches
Femoral Vein + tributaries
Superficial Inguinal Lymph Nodes + tributaries (Superolateral, Superomedial + Inguinal)
Deep Iliac Lymph Nodes + tributaries

Considerations of abdominal/pelvic structures that are taken off of tension during flexion of the leg.

Lumbar Plexus
Sympathetic Trunk
Celiac Plexus
Superior Mesenteric Plexus
Inferior Mesenteric Plexus
Suprarenal + Renal Plexus
Ovarian/Testicular Plexus
Superior + Inferior Hypogastric Plexus
Abdominal Aorta, Internal/External Iliac Artery + branches
Inferior Vena Cava + tributaries
Ascending Lumbar Veins + tributaries
Cisterna chyli
Lymph Trunks
Epigastric Lymph Nodes
Splenic Lymph Nodes
Lumbar Lymph Nodes + tributaries
Superior Mesenteric Lymph Nodes + tributaries
Inferior Mesenteric Lymph Nodes + tributaries
Common Iliac Lymph Nodes + tributaries
External Iliac Lymph Nodes + tributaries
Internal Iliac Lymph Nodes + tributaries
Peritoneum
Mesenteries
Visceral Field

Abdominal Field
Bringing the leg into flexion during leg rotations places the ventral tissues and neurovascular structures on slack.

Inguinal Area
Rotation of the leg brings the structures in the inguinal area on and off of compression by changing the position of the bony framework and muscular tensions of the leg.

The on/off tension and slack of the soft tissues encourages the movement of fluids within the vascular structures and lymph nodes.

* The above charts demonstrate only a sampling of structures that may be affected during a leg rotation.

FIG 3.23

Anatomy of the Leg Rotation: Flexion Considerations of Dorsal Structures

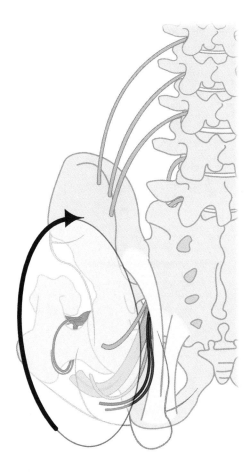

Considerations of dorsal structures affected during flexion of the leg.

Superior Cluneal Nerves
Sciatic Nerve (L4-S3)
Inferior Gluteal Nerve (L5-S2) + branches
Posterior Femoral Cutaneous Nerve (S1-S3) + branches
Anterior Spinal Artery + branches
Posterior Spinal Artery + branches
Inferior Gluteal Artery
Medial Circumflex Artery
Batson Venous Plexus
Internal Vertebral Venous Plexus
Anterior Spinal Vein + tributaries
Posterior Spinal Vein + tributaries
Posterolateral Spinal Vein + tributaries
Inferior Gluteal Vein
Medial Circumflex Femoral Vein
Lymphatic Capillaries
Spinal cord + meninges

* The above chart demonstrates only a sampling of structures that may be affected during a leg rotation.

Dorsal Considerations for Flexion

Bringing the leg into flexion during leg rotations places the dorsal tissues on tension as the pelvis tips posterior, pulling the soft tissue over the ischial tuberosity.

Bringing the leg into a flexed position lengthens the dorsal line of the body, causing unilateral flexion on the same side and lengthening the corresponding dorsal tissues.

FIG 3.24

Anatomy of the Leg Rotation: Considerations of Structures Affected by the Medial Arc

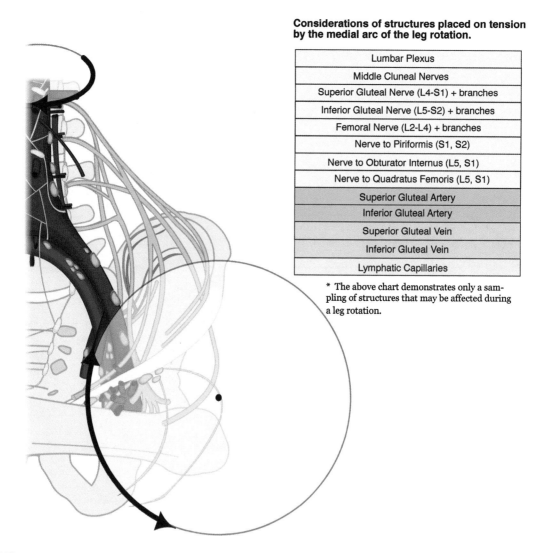

Considerations of structures placed on tension by the medial arc of the leg rotation.

Lumbar Plexus
Middle Cluneal Nerves
Superior Gluteal Nerve (L4-S1) + branches
Inferior Gluteal Nerve (L5-S2) + branches
Femoral Nerve (L2-L4) + branches
Nerve to Piriformis (S1, S2)
Nerve to Obturator Internus (L5, S1)
Nerve to Quadratus Femoris (L5, S1)
Superior Gluteal Artery
Inferior Gluteal Artery
Superior Gluteal Vein
Inferior Gluteal Vein
Lymphatic Capillaries

* The above chart demonstrates only a sampling of structures that may be affected during a leg rotation.

Dorsal Tissues
Tissues on the dorsal side of the abdomen and pelvis of the ipsilateral side are generally placed on tension during the medial arc of a leg rotation.

Abdominal Field
Guiding the leg into the medial arc of a leg rotation brings the soft tissue of the abdomen on slack.

SI Joint and Lumbar Facets
Effect of medial arc of the leg rotation on the SI joint and lumbar vertebrae:
  • SI joint opens
  • Facets on the side of the leg rotation unilaterally close; the corresponding facet on the contralateral side will open (side-bending and rotation).

Inguinal Area & Pelvic Floor
Tissues and structures in the inguinal fold are placed under compression during the medial arc of the leg rotation. Tissues of the pelvic floor are slackened.

FIG 3.25

Anatomy of the Leg Rotation: Considerations of Structures Affected by the Lateral Arc

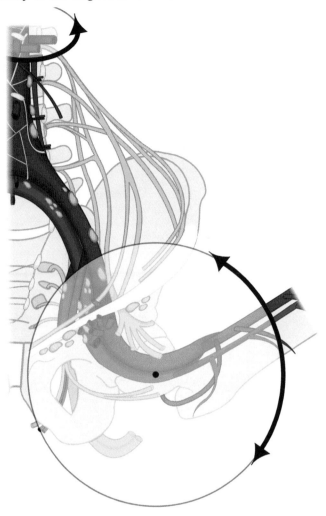

Considerations of structures placed on tension by the lateral arc of the leg rotation.

Celiac Plexus
Superior Mesenteric Plexus
Inferior Mesenteric Plexus
Suprarenal + Renal Plexus
Ovarian/Testicular Plexus
Superior + Inferior Hypogastric Plexus
Femoral Nerve (L2-L4) + branches
Obturator Nerve (L2-L4) + branches
Abdominal Aorta, Internal/External Iliac Artery + branches
Femoral Artery + branches
Obturator Artery + branches
Internal Pudendal Artery + branches
Inferior Vena Cava, Internal/ External Iliac Vein + tributaries
Ascending Lumbar Veins + tributaries
Femoral Vein + tributaries
Obturator Vein
Internal Pudendal Vein + tributaries
Cisterna chyli
Lymph Trunks
Epigastric Lymph Nodes
Splenic Lymph Nodes
Lumbar Lymph Nodes + tributaries
Superior Mesenteric Lymph Nodes + tributaries
Inferior Mesenteric Lymph Nodes + tributaries
Common Iliac Lymph Nodes + tributaries
External Iliac Lymph Nodes + tributaries
Internal Iliac Lymph Nodes + tributaries
Peritoneum
Mesenteries
Visceral Field

* The above chart demonstrates only a sampling of structures that may be affected during a leg rotation.

Dorsal Tissues
Tissues on the dorsal side of the abdomen and pelvis of the ipsilateral side are generally slackened during the lateral arc of a leg rotation.

Abdominal Field
Guiding the leg into the lateral arc of a leg rotation brings the soft tissue of the abdomen on tension.

SI Joint and Lumbar Facets
Effect of lateral arc of the leg rotation on the SI joint and lumbar vertebrae:
  • SI joint closes
  • Facets on the side of the leg rotation unilaterally open; the corresponding facet on the contralateral side will close (rotation and side-bending).

Inguinal Area & Pelvic Floor
Force from the lateral arc of the leg rotation can adjust to place tension on the inguinal area or pelvic floor.

FIG 3.26

Anatomy of the Leg Rotation: Lumbar Plexus (Sites of potential obstruction)

Iliohypogastric Nerve (L1)

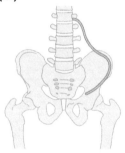
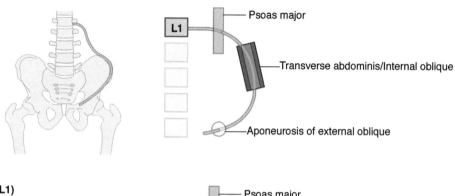

Ilioinguinal Nerve (L1)

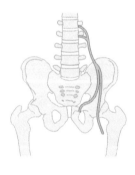
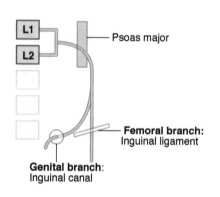

Genitofemoral Nerve (L1-L2)

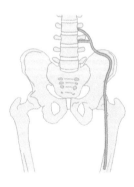
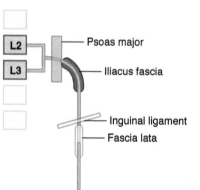

Lateral Femoral Cutaneous Nerve (L2-L3)

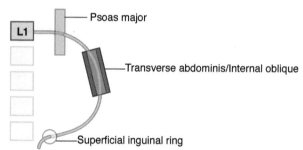

FIG 3.27 (a)

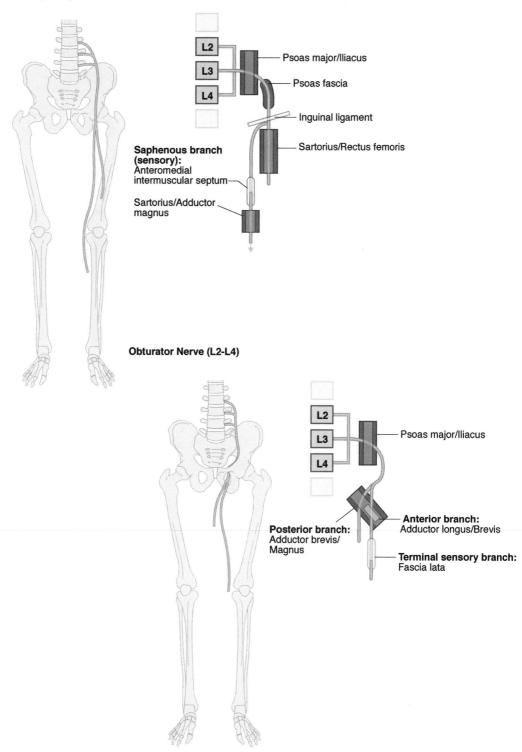

Femoral Nerve (L2-L4)

L2
L3
L4

Psoas major/Iliacus

Psoas fascia

Inguinal ligament

Sartorius/Rectus femoris

Saphenous branch (sensory):
Anteromedial intermuscular septum

Sartorius/Adductor magnus

Obturator Nerve (L2-L4)

L2
L3
L4

Psoas major/Iliacus

Posterior branch:
Adductor brevis/Magnus

Anterior branch:
Adductor longus/Brevis

Terminal sensory branch:
Fascia lata

FIG 3.27 (b)

Anatomy of the Leg Rotation: Sacral Plexus (Sites of potential obstruction)

Superior Gluteal Nerve (L4-S1)

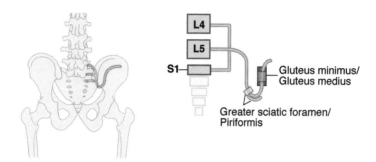

Inferior Gluteal Nerve (L5-S2)

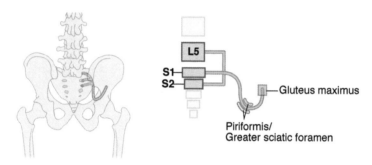

Posterior Femoral Cutaneous Nerve (S1-S3)

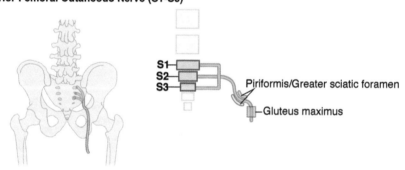

Pudendal Nerve (S2-S4)

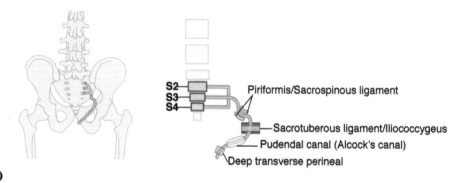

FIG 3.28 (a)

Sciatic Nerve (L4-S3)

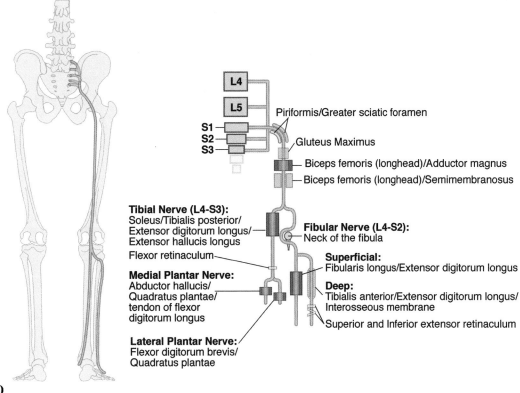

L4

L5

S1
S2
S3

Piriformis/Greater sciatic foramen

Gluteus Maximus

Biceps femoris (longhead)/Adductor magnus

Biceps femoris (longhead)/Semimembranosus

Tibial Nerve (L4-S3):
Soleus/Tibialis posterior/
Extensor digitorum longus/
Extensor hallucis longus

Flexor retinaculum

Medial Plantar Nerve:
Abductor hallucis/
Quadratus plantae/
tendon of flexor
digitorum longus

Lateral Plantar Nerve:
Flexor digitorum brevis/
Quadratus plantae

Fibular Nerve (L4-S2):
Neck of the fibula

Superficial:
Fibularis longus/Extensor digitorum longus

Deep:
Tibialis anterior/Extensor digitorum longus/
Interosseous membrane

Superior and Inferior extensor retinaculum

FIG 3.28 (b)

Anatomy of the Leg Rotation: Pelvic Arteries (Sites of potential obstruction)

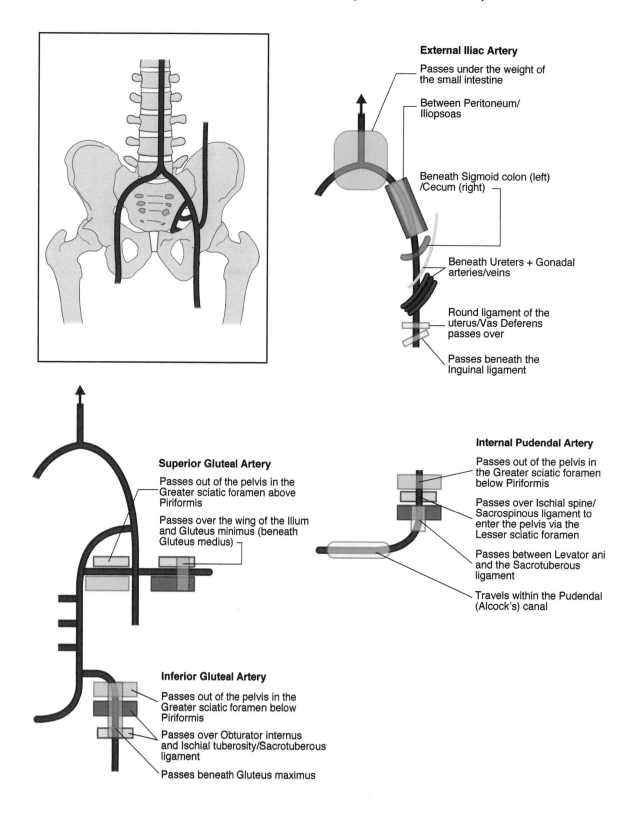

External Iliac Artery

Passes under the weight of the small intestine

Between Peritoneum/ Iliopsoas

Beneath Sigmoid colon (left) /Cecum (right)

Beneath Ureters + Gonadal arteries/veins

Round ligament of the uterus/Vas Deferens passes over

Passes beneath the Inguinal ligament

Superior Gluteal Artery

Passes out of the pelvis in the Greater sciatic foramen above Piriformis

Passes over the wing of the Ilium and Gluteus minimus (beneath Gluteus medius)

Internal Pudendal Artery

Passes out of the pelvis in the Greater sciatic foramen below Piriformis

Passes over Ischial spine/ Sacrospinous ligament to enter the pelvis via the Lesser sciatic foramen

Passes between Levator ani and the Sacrotuberous ligament

Travels within the Pudendal (Alcock's) canal

Inferior Gluteal Artery

Passes out of the pelvis in the Greater sciatic foramen below Piriformis

Passes over Obturator internus and Ischial tuberosity/Sacrotuberous ligament

Passes beneath Gluteus maximus

FIG 3.29   * Note: Not all arteries of the pelvis are represented.

Anatomy of the Leg Rotation: Pelvic Veins (Sites of potential obstruction)

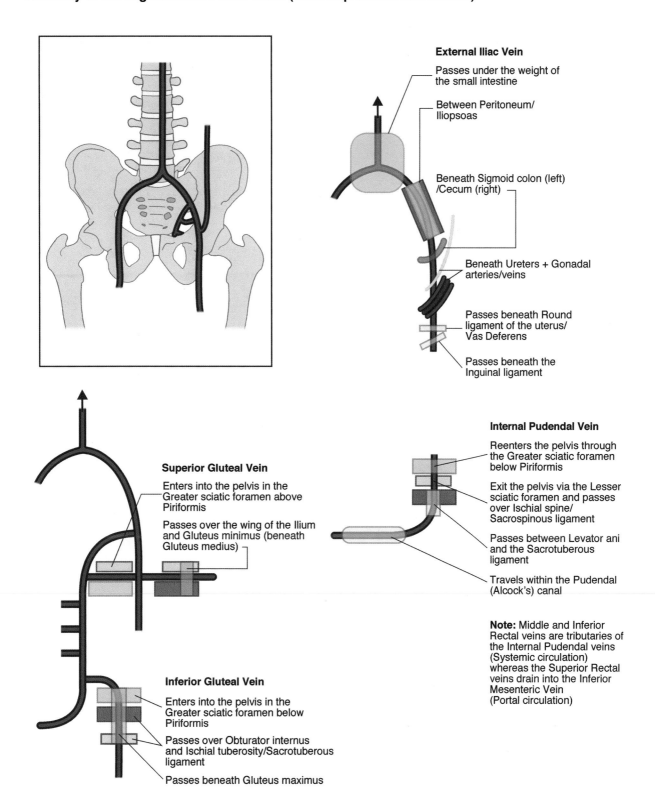

External Iliac Vein

Passes under the weight of the small intestine

Between Peritoneum/ Iliopsoas

Beneath Sigmoid colon (left) /Cecum (right)

Beneath Ureters + Gonadal arteries/veins

Passes beneath Round ligament of the uterus/ Vas Deferens

Passes beneath the Inguinal ligament

Superior Gluteal Vein

Enters into the pelvis in the Greater sciatic foramen above Piriformis

Passes over the wing of the Ilium and Gluteus minimus (beneath Gluteus medius)

Inferior Gluteal Vein

Enters into the pelvis in the Greater sciatic foramen below Piriformis

Passes over Obturator internus and Ischial tuberosity/Sacrotuberous ligament

Passes beneath Gluteus maximus

Internal Pudendal Vein

Reenters the pelvis through the Greater sciatic foramen below Piriformis

Exit the pelvis via the Lesser sciatic foramen and passes over Ischial spine/ Sacrospinous ligament

Passes between Levator ani and the Sacrotuberous ligament

Travels within the Pudendal (Alcock's) canal

Note: Middle and Inferior Rectal veins are tributaries of the Internal Pudendal veins (Systemic circulation) whereas the Superior Rectal veins drain into the Inferior Mesenteric Vein (Portal circulation)

FIG 3.30   * Note: Not all veins of the pelvis are represented.

Anatomy of the Leg Rotation: Arteries of the Lower Extremity (Sites of potential obstruction)

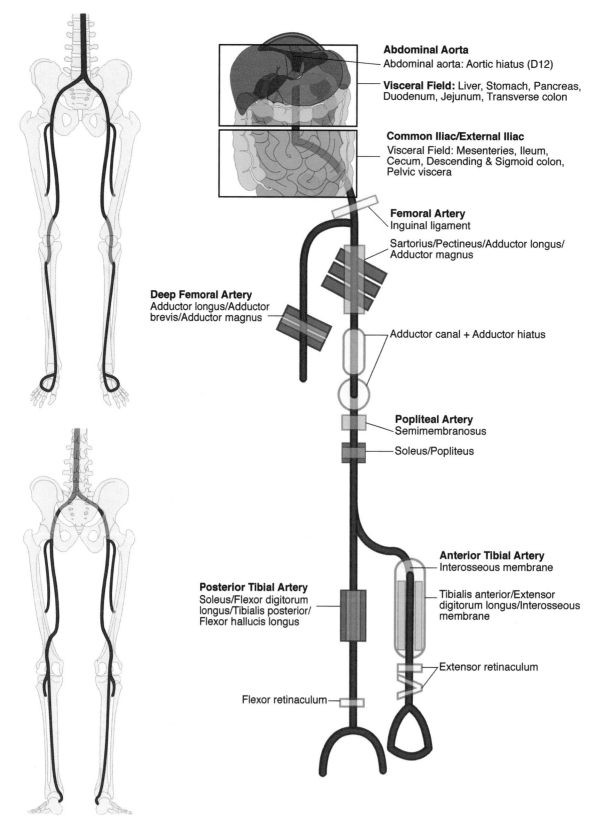

Abdominal Aorta
Abdominal aorta: Aortic hiatus (D12)

Visceral Field: Liver, Stomach, Pancreas, Duodenum, Jejunum, Transverse colon

Common Iliac/External Iliac
Visceral Field: Mesenteries, Ileum, Cecum, Descending & Sigmoid colon, Pelvic viscera

Femoral Artery
Inguinal ligament

Sartorius/Pectineus/Adductor longus/ Adductor magnus

Deep Femoral Artery
Adductor longus/Adductor brevis/Adductor magnus

Adductor canal + Adductor hiatus

Popliteal Artery
Semimembranosus

Soleus/Popliteus

Anterior Tibial Artery
Interosseous membrane

Tibialis anterior/Extensor digitorum longus/Interosseous membrane

Posterior Tibial Artery
Soleus/Flexor digitorum longus/Tibialis posterior/ Flexor hallucis longus

Extensor retinaculum

Flexor retinaculum

FIG 3.31

* Note: Not all arteries of the lower extremity are represented.

Anatomy of the Leg Rotation: Veins of the Lower Extremity (Sites of potential obstruction)

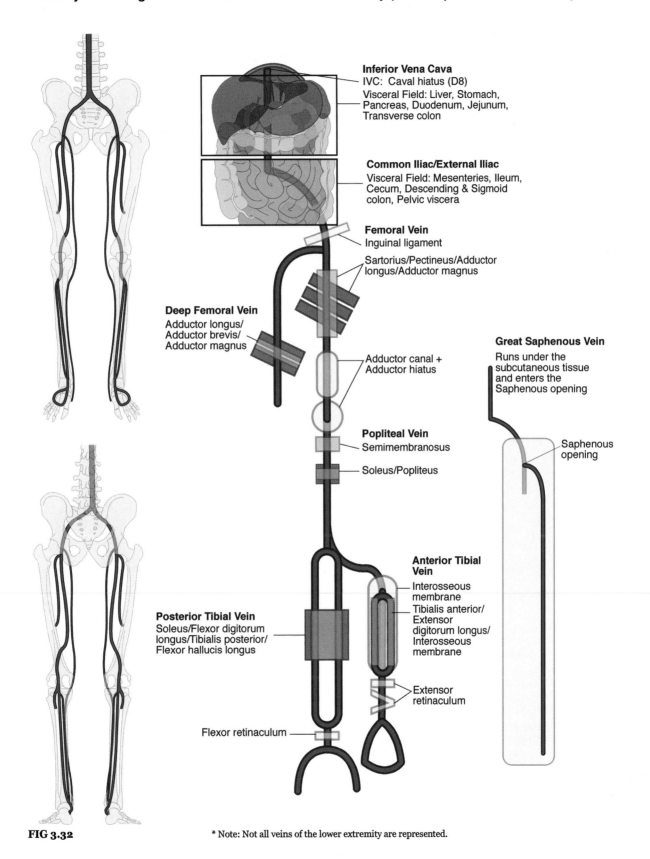

Inferior Vena Cava
IVC: Caval hiatus (D8)
Visceral Field: Liver, Stomach, Pancreas, Duodenum, Jejunum, Transverse colon

Common Iliac/External Iliac
Visceral Field: Mesenteries, Ileum, Cecum, Descending & Sigmoid colon, Pelvic viscera

Femoral Vein
Inguinal ligament

Sartorius/Pectineus/Adductor longus/Adductor magnus

Deep Femoral Vein
Adductor longus/
Adductor brevis/
Adductor magnus

Adductor canal +
Adductor hiatus

Great Saphenous Vein

Runs under the subcutaneous tissue and enters the Saphenous opening

Saphenous opening

Popliteal Vein
Semimembranosus

Soleus/Popliteus

Anterior Tibial Vein
Interosseous membrane
Tibialis anterior/
Extensor digitorum longus/
Interosseous membrane

Posterior Tibial Vein
Soleus/Flexor digitorum longus/Tibialis posterior/
Flexor hallucis longus

Extensor retinaculum

Flexor retinaculum

FIG 3.32

* Note: Not all veins of the lower extremity are represented.

Anatomy of the Leg Rotation: Lymphatics of the Lower Extremity (Sites of potential obstruction)

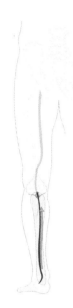

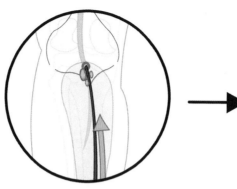

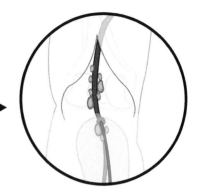

Superficial Lymphatic Drainage of Posterolateral Leg

To superficial popliteal lymph nodes accompanying the small saphenous vein.

Path: Superficial Drainage of Posterolateral leg

The lymph from the superficial posterolateral leg passes through:

• Posterior compartment fascia
• Medial and lateral heads of gastrocnemius

Path: Deep Drainage of Posterolateral leg

The lymphatic fluid from the superficial lymph nodes of the leg and foot travels to the deep popliteal lymph nodes. Accompanying the popliteal vein, the lymph passes under:

• Biceps Femoris and semimembranosus

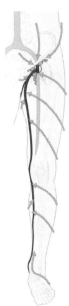

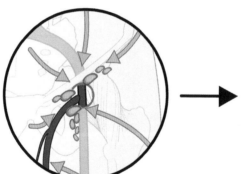

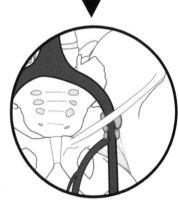

Superficial Lymphatic Drainage of Lower Extremity

Superficial lymphatic drainage of the lower extremity predominantly travels to the superficial inguinal lymph nodes (Inferior inguinal, superomedial & superolateral).

Path: Superficial Drainage of the Lower Extremity

The lymph from the superficial lower extremity (excluding the posterolateral leg, described above), passes from the superficial inguinal lymph nodes to the deep inguinal lymph nodes. The lymph passes through:

• Saphenous opening

Path: Deep Drainage of Lower Extremity

The lymph from the superficial inguinal lymph nodes, the deep popliteal lymph nodes and the lymph from deep structures (ie. muscles, joints and nerves), drains into the deep inguinal lymph nodes. The lymph passes through:

• Inguinal ligament

FIG 3·33

Cisterna Chyli + Thoracic Duct

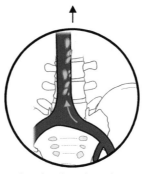

Lumbar lymph nodes

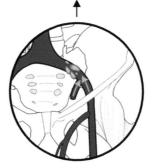

Common Iliac lymph nodes

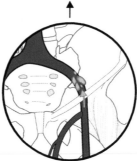

External Iliac lymph nodes

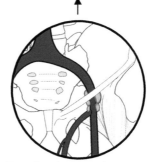

Deep Inguinal lymph nodes

Respiratory Diaphragm

The respiratory diaphragm has implications in arterial, venous, and lymphatic circulation and contains crucial nervous structures coursing through to the abdominal viscera. As such, ensuring that the diaphragm is capable of moving through its entire range of motion is of utmost importance for every area of the body.

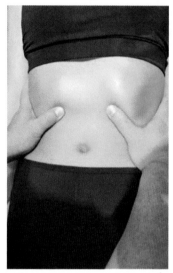

FIG 3.34: *Assessing motion of the diaphragm.*

To assess the motion of the diaphragm, the operator takes hold below the inferior angle of the rib cage at the costochondral margin and splays his thumbs on the medial edge of the costal cartilage (**FIG 3.34**). It is important to note that, upon initial palpation, this area will likely feel asymmetrical from left to right, especially at its most medial aspect. This asymmetry is due to the location of the viscera: the right side feels more full owing to the presence of the liver (the stomach, which is generally less substantial, is on the left). These variations should not be mistakenly diagnosed as a lesion per se. Upon inhalation operators should palpate a global excursion of the bony framework into their hands, as well as an accompanied descent of the diaphragm at their thumbs. During this inhalation the operator can use his thumbs as fixed points between which the diaphragm must descend and narrow, thus treating the soft muscular tissue of the diaphragm. Upon exhalation the operator can follow the diaphragm in its ascent and gently encourage its motion upwards, a process sometimes referred to as 'doming' the diaphragm, with his thumb pads (**FIG 3.35**).

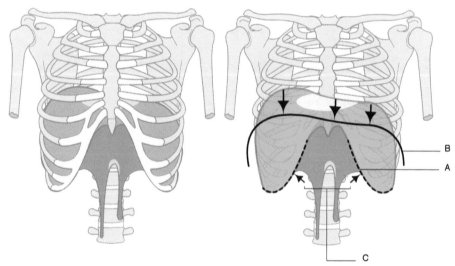

FIG 3.35: *Doming the diaphragm.* The operator can assess the descent of the diaphragm during inhalation. Palpating along the inferior angle of the rib cage (a), the diaphragm will descend upon inhalation (b); upon exhalation the operator can follow the diaphragm in its ascent and encourage motion upwards with his thumb pads (c).

To further investigate the ribs more focally and thus obtain a better diagnosis of the diaphragm, the operator can palpate the interspaces between ribs (**FIG 3.36, 3.37**), meaning that the operator places his hands such that the actual rib is between his fingers. Upon inhalation there should be an element of gapping between ribs, whereas upon exhalation there should be a narrowing of the interspace. Should the operator palpate an asymmetry or restriction in motion (while keeping with the base-up, centre-out principle), diagnosis and treatment of the thoracic spine should precede treatment of the ribs themselves.

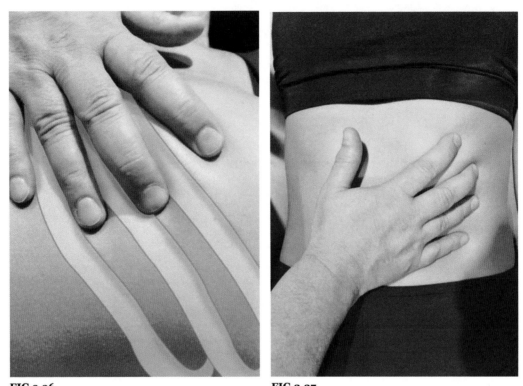

FIG 3.36   **FIG 3.37**

Diagnosing the diaphragm via palpation of the intercostal spaces.

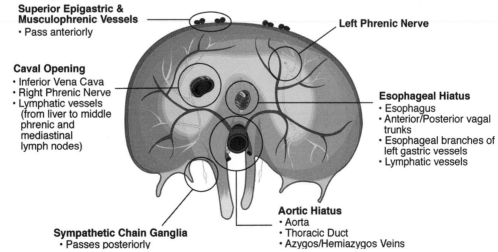

FIG 3.38: *An example of notable structures passing through the respiratory diaphragm.*

Anatomy of the Respiratory Diaphragm: Related Viscera

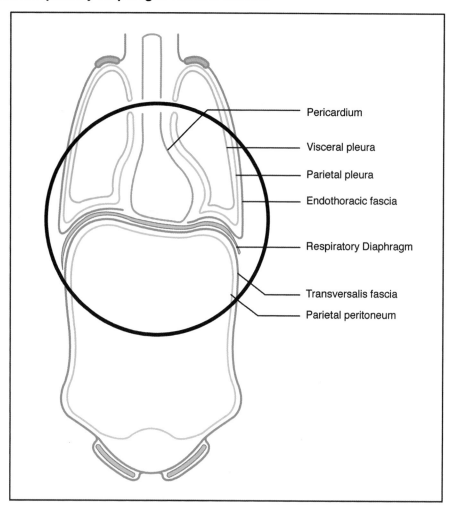

Pericardium

Visceral pleura

Parietal pleura

Endothoracic fascia

Respiratory Diaphragm

Transversalis fascia

Parietal peritoneum

THORACIC VISCERA

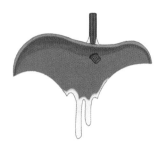

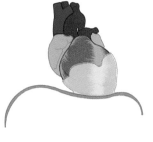

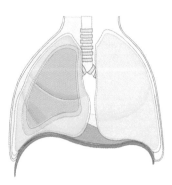

Esophagus
• Attachment to the diaphragm via the phrenoesophageal ligaments
• Passes through the diaphragm at T10

Heart
• Attachment to the diaphragm via the fibrous pericardium

Lungs
• Attachment to the diaphragm via the endothoracic fascia/ parietal pleura

FIG 3.39 (a)

ABDOMINAL VISCERA

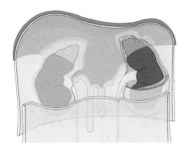

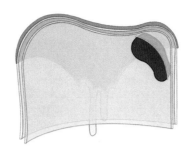

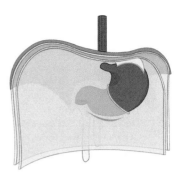

Kidneys
- Attachment to diaphragm via the renal fascia that blends into the diaphragmatic fascia
- The kidneys are retroperitoneal

Spleen
- Attachment to the diaphragm via the splenophrenic ligament
- Due to its location directly inferior to it, the spleen is affected by the mobility of the diaphragm
- The spleen is intraperitoneal

Stomach
- Attachment to the diaphragm via the gastrophrenic ligament
- Affected by the attachment to the liver via the gastrohepatic ligament
- The stomach is intraperitoneal

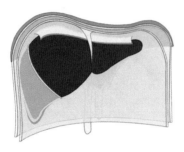

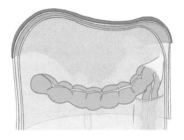

Liver
- Attachment to the diaphragm via the falciform ligament, coronary ligament & triangular ligament
- The liver is intraperitoneal

Splenic Flexure of Colon
- Attachment to the diaphragm via the phrenicocolic ligament
- The descending colon is retroperitoneal in most people

FIG 3.39 (b)

Three Cardinal Arm Movements

The three cardinal arm movements are used as a baseline diagnosis to explore motion of the clavicle upon the first rib in all three planes: sagittal, coronal, and transverse. The motion of the clavicle is important for many reasons, one reason being the presence of essential neurovascular structures that travel from the superior thoracic aperture and cervical spine into the upper limbs. The movements can also be used as a form of diagnosis for the upper T-line, and as preparation for the treatment of the superior thoracic aperture.

First Cardinal Arm Movement

The first movement explores motion of the clavicle as it lifts off of the chest wall in a sagittal plane. With a straight body position, the operator cups the patient's wrist around the carpals and holds the arm against the his body, just lateral to his own midline, with the outside hand. This ensures that the patient will move along with the operator as he uses his own body to induce motion, using the arm as a lever, through to the patient's clavicle. As with all osteopathic treatment, this hold will vary from patient to patient and operator to operator; in certain circumstances the operator may find it beneficial to use a forearm-to-forearm grasping method, or even bend the patient's arm at the elbow to create a hook from which to hold. Although the hold will vary, of utmost importance is that the operator is able to execute control of the lever and create leverage all the way to the fixed point with the exe-

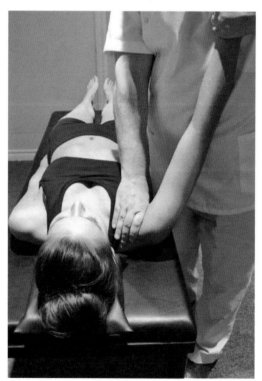 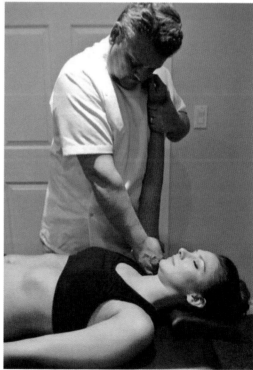

FIG 3.40   **FIG 3.41**

Using the first cardinal arm movement to assess the glenohumeral or scapulothoracic joints.

cution of correct body mechanics and rhythm.

Once the operator has full control of the patient's arm, he can use it and his remaining hand as a tool in diagnosis (via palpation and treatment) by creating a fixed point. For example, the operator can cup around the glenohumeral joint (**FIG 3.40, 3.41**) and assess how much resistance is encountered as the entire scapulothoracic girdle is lifted off the table, or he can palpate along the clavicular joints to assess the motion capabilities. By comparing this assessment to that of the patient's other shoulder, the operator will gain an understanding of the overall torsion within the patient's lesion pattern.

To bring motion to the clavicle using the arm in a sagittal plane, the operator stands in a fencer stance whereby one leg is ahead of the other, and feet are pointing in the direction the operator is facing. The operator shifts weight from one foot to the other in a rhythmical, rocking motion; as the operator executes this motion, he guides the patient's arm in a pendulum-like movement. During this motion, the operator can place his thumb pad directly beneath the clavicle, beginning midline at the sternal end (**FIG 3.42**), and follow along the line beneath the clavicle laterally towards the acromial end (**FIG 3.43**). It is important that the operator palpate at their thumb pad while maintaining a flat hand with a broad contact on the opposite side of the patient's chest. This particular positioning of the hand will help to control the opposite shoulder, similar to how their hand was used to control the opposite hip during a leg rotation in supine position (namely, to ensure that motion can be controlled within the area being assessed). This movement assesses the mobility of the clavicle off of the first ribs, particularly during motion in the sagittal plane and rotation of the upper T-line about a vertical axis. Bear in mind, though, that this assessment can also be applied to the upper ribs, whose primary motion likewise originates in the sagittal plane. To assess motion of the ribs in this position, the operator simply moves a palpatory hand to the anterior aspect of the ribs during this first cardinal arm movement.

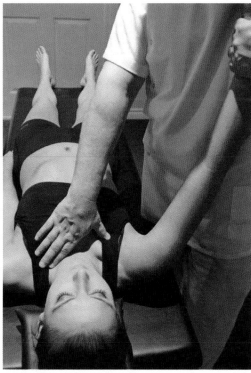 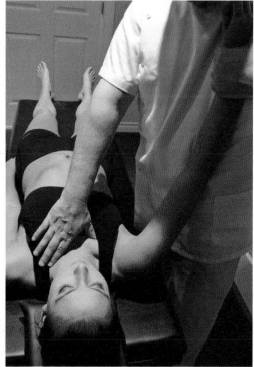

FIG 3.42   **FIG 3.43**

Using the first cardinal arm movement to assess motion of the clavicle in the sagittal plane.

Anatomy of the First Cardinal Arm Movement: Musculature

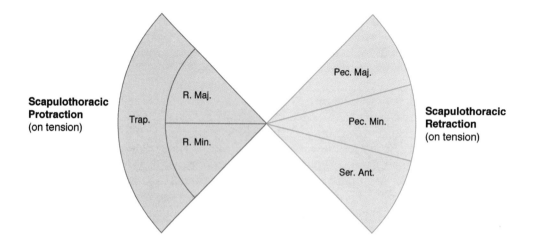

Scapulothoracic Protraction

Muscle	Origin	Insertion	Innervation
Trapezius	Nuchal line of the occiput, nuchal ligament, and SPs of the dorsal spine	Lateral third of the clavicle, acromion, and scapular spine in three portions (descending, transverse, and ascending)	CNXI Spinal Accessory and cervical spinal nerves C2-C4
Rhomboid Major & Minor	Nuchal ligament and SPs of C7-T1 (minor) and T2-T5 (major)	Medial border of the scapula	Dorsal scapular nerve (C4, C5)

Scapulothoracic Retraction

Muscle	Origin	Insertion	Innervation
Pectoralis Major	Sternal end of the clavicle and the sternocostal joints of ribs 1-7	Greater tubercle of the humerus	Medial (C8-T1) and lateral pectoral (C5-C7)
Pectoralis Minor	Coracoid process	Ribs 3-5	
Serratus Anterior	Ventral surface of the scapula	Lateral surface of ribs 1-8	Long Thoracic (C5-C7)

FIG 3.44

Anatomy of the First Cardinal Arm Movement: Considerations of Structures Affected

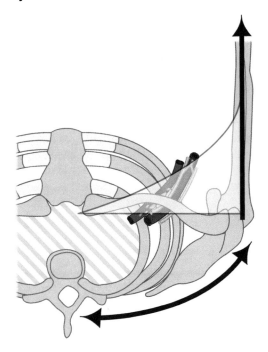

Protraction

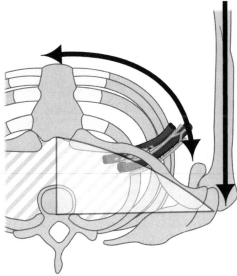

Retraction

FIG 3.45

Considerations of structures affected by first cardinal arm movement.

Brachial Plexus
Phrenic Nerve (C3-C5)
Vagus Nerve (CN X)
Recurrent Laryngeal
First Thoracic Nerves
Sympathetic Chains
Brachiocephalic Artery + branches
Left Subclavian Artery + branches
Superior Intercostal Arteries
Internal Thoracic Arteries
Dorsal Scapular Arteries
Subscapular Arteries
Brachiocephalic Vein + tributaries
Subclavian Vein + tributaries
Dorsal Scapular Vein + tributaries
Subscapular Vein + tributaries
Thoracic Ducts
Subclavian Lymph Trunks
Axillary Lymph Nodes
Pectoral Lymph Nodes
Subscapular Lymph Nodes
Sibson's Fascia
Visceral Field

* The above chart demonstrates only a sampling of structures that may be affected.

PROTRACTION

Clavicle
Using the arm as a long lever, the operator lifts the clavicle off of the first rib, freeing the neurovascular tissue passing to the upper extremity.

Thorax
Using the arm as a lever the operator may encourage rotation on the contralateral side. The operator may consider a fulcrum to affect the ribcage, encouraging selected ribs anteriorly.

Tissue
Tissue along the posterior aspect of the shoulder girdle is placed on tension while tissue on the anterior aspect is placed on slack.

RETRACTION

Thorax

Using the arm as a lever the operator may encourage rotation on the ipsilateral side. The operator may consider a fulcrum to affect the ribcage, encouraging selected ribs posteriorly.

Tissue
Tissue along the anterior aspect of the shoulder girdle is place on tension while tissue on the posterior aspect is placed on slack.

Second Cardinal Arm Movement

The second cardinal arm movement carries the same principles as the first, and takes into account the operator's stance, body mechanics and rhythm. However, the motion of the lever, and thus the motion of the clavicle, change in tandem. The operator switches his hold of the arm from his outside hand to the inside hand, grasping just beneath the elbow joint to extend—while careful not to hyperextend—the lever against his body and straighten the arm. The rocking motion from foot to foot is the same but for one exception: the motion that is induced by the position of the lever, which is one of sidebending within the coronal plane, rotates around an anterior/posterior axis. The operator's outside hand now becomes the palpatory tool to assess cephalad/caudad glide of the clavicle off of the chest wall, again beginning at midline and moving laterally (**FIG 3.46, 3.47**). This creates sidebending of the scapulothoracic girdle and, similar to how the first cardinal arm movement assessed rotation of the upper T-line, this movement assesses sidebending of the upper T-line. At this point, operators should be taking note of how their findings in this position correlate to the findings from the first movement.

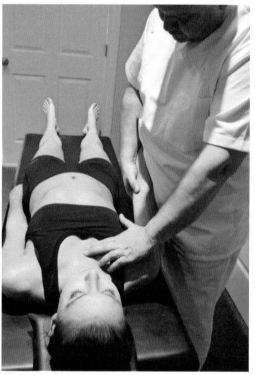 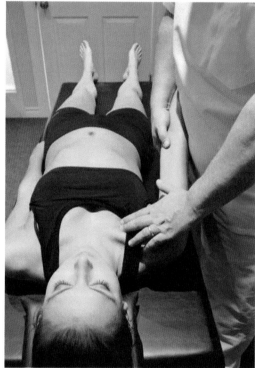

FIG 3.46   **FIG 3.47**

Using the second cardinal arm movement to assess motion of the clavicle in the coronal plane.

Anatomy of the Second Cardinal Arm Movement: Musculature

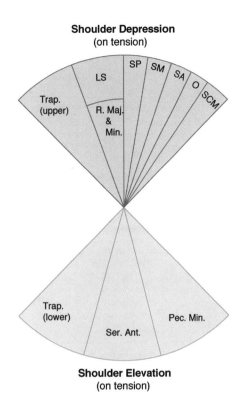

Shoulder Elevation			
Muscle	**Origin**	**Insertion**	**Innervation**
Trapezius	Nuchal line of the occiput, nuchal ligament, and SPs of the dorsal spine	Lateral third of the clavicle, acromion, and scapular spine in three portions (descending, transverse, and ascending)	CNXI Spinal Accessory and cervical spinal nerves C2-C4
Serratus Anterior	Ventral surface of the scapula	Lateral surface of ribs 1-8	Long Thoracic (C5-C7)
Pectoralis Minor	Coracoid process	Ribs 3-5	Medial (C8-T1) and lateral pectoral (C5-C7)

FIG 3.48(a)

Shoulder Depression			
Muscle	**Origin**	**Insertion**	**Innervation**
Trapezius	Nuchal line of the occiput, nuchal ligament, and SPs of the dorsal spine	Lateral third of the clavicle, acromion, and scapular spine in three portions (descending, transverse, and ascending)	CNXI Spinal Accessory and cervical spinal nerves C2-C4
Levator Scapulae	TPs of C1-C4	Superior medial border of the scapula	Dorsal scapular nerve (C4, C5)
Rhomboid Major & Minor	Nuchal ligament and SPs of C7-T1 (minor) and T2-T5 (major)	Medial border of the scapula	Dorsal scapular nerve (C4, C5)
Scalene Posterior	Posterior tubercles C4-C6	Rib 2	Cervical spinal nerves and brachial plexus
Scalene Middle	Posterior tubercles C2-C7	Rib 1	
Scalene Anterior	Anterior tubercles C3-C6	Rib 1	
Omohyoid	Hyoid	Superior border of the scapula via a superior and inferior belly	Ansa cervicalis, inferior trunk (C1-C3)
SCM	Mastoid process and nuchal line	Manubrium and clavicle	CNXI Spinal Accessory (C1-C6) and cervical spinal nerves

FIG 3.48(b)

Anatomy of the Second Cardinal Arm Movement: Considerations of Structures Affected

DEPRESSION

Supraclavicular/Neck
Using the arm as a long lever, and inducing sidebending to the upper T-line the operator places ipsilateral tissues of the neck on tension.

Clavicle
Sidebending of the upper T-line may decrease the size of passage for the neurovascular structures passing below.

ELEVATION

Supraclavicular/Neck
Using the arm as a long lever and bringing it superior will place the ipsilateral tissues of the neck on slack.

Clavicle
Bringing the arm superior opens the subclavicular area, potentially freeing the neurovascular structures below.

Thorax
Tissue and neurovascular structures through the upper and mid thorax are placed on tension.

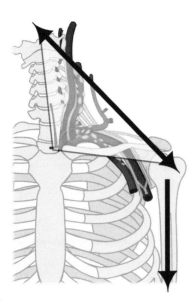

Depression

Considerations of structures placed on tension by depression of the upper T-line.

Brachial Plexus
Cervical Plexus
Glossopharyngeal Nerve (CN IX)
Vagus Nerve (CN X)
Accessory Nerve (CN XI)
Hypoglossal Nerve (CN XII)
Cervical Ganglia
Subclavian Artery + branches
Common Carotid Artery + branches
Subclavian Vein + tributaries
Inferior Thyroid Vein
Superficial Lymph Nodes of the Neck + tributaries
Submental Lymph Nodes + tributaries
Submandibular Lymph Nodes + tributaries
Deep Cervical Lymph Nodes + tributaries
Anterior Cervical Lymph Nodes + tributaries
Investing Fascia
Prevertebral Fascia
Pretracheal Fascia
Visceral Field

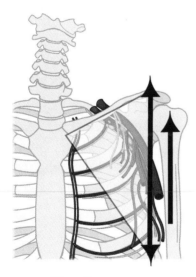

Elevation

Considerations of structures placed on tension by elevation of the upper T-line.

Long Thoracic Nerve (C5-C7)
Cervical Plexus
Lateral/Medial Pectoral Nerve
Thoracodorsal Nerve (C6-C8)
Intercostal Nerves
Superior Thoracic Artery
Pectoral branch of the Thoracoacromial A.
Lateral Thoracic Artery
Subscapular Artery + branches
Intercostal Arteries
Thoracoacromial Vein + tributaries
Lateral Thoracic Vein
Thoracoepigastric Vein + tributaries
Subscapular Vein + tributaries
Intercostal Veins
Superficial Lymph Vessels of the Thoracic wall
Visceral Field

* The above charts demonstrate only a sampling of structures that may be affected.

FIG 3.49

Third Cardinal Arm Movement

The third cardinal arm movement, which carries the same principles as the first two, assesses motion of the clavicle as it rotates anteriorly/posteriorly upon the first rib (**FIG 3.50, 3.51**). The operator can approach the movement from above or below the arm facing downtable or uptable, respectively, so long as the principles of leverage, rhythm, and body mechanics are applied correctly. The operator switches the hand hold such that he again holds the patient's arm in his outside hand, grasping as near to the elbow as possible. The operator must bring the patient's arm into enough abduction in the coronal plane so that tension is built at the clavicle; at this point, the inside hand has now become the palpatory hand, which moves along the clavicle. Once this tension is reached, the operator then rotates the arm in a counter-clockwise direction, utilizing the inertia of the arm to rotate the clavicle. The hold must be soft so that the shoulder girdle is able to find its own glide pattern. If operators steer the arm instead of allowing it to move in its own motion capacity, they run the risk of injuring the patient, as a motion has been imposed onto a joint that is beyond the focus of this movement. Remember that because the palpatory hand is at the clavicle, the restriction is felt at the clavicle in its anterior/posterior rotation rather than in the rotation of the lever (the humeral head within the glenoid fossa). This lever is simply acting as a crank to generate and transfer tension to exert motion at the clavicle. This third cardinal arm movement aims to balance the upper T-line anteriorly/posteriorly on a transverse plane as well as through rotation of the upper T-line about a vertical axis.

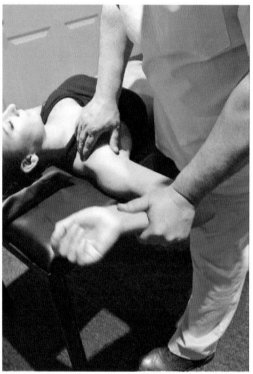
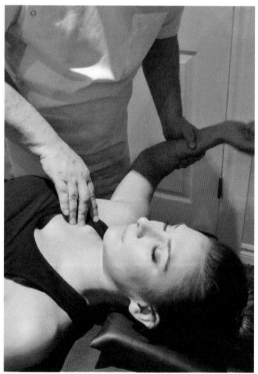

FIG 3.50   **FIG 3.51**

Using the third cardinal arm movement to assess motion of the clavicle in the transverse plane.

Anatomy of the Third Cardinal Arm Movement: Musculature

**Glenohumeral
External Rotation
(on tension)**

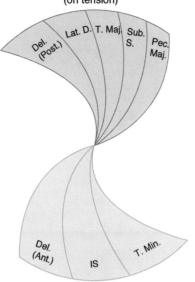

**Glenohumeral
Internal Rotation
(on tension)**

Glenohumeral External Rotation			
Muscle	**Origin**	**Insertion**	**Innervation**
Deltoid	Lateral third of the clavicle, acromion, and scapular spine	Deltoid tuberosity of the humerus	Axillary (C5-C6)
Latissimus Dorsi	SPs of T6-T12, thoracolumbar fascia, iliac crest, and lower 4 ribs	Inferior angle of the scapula and intertubercular groove of the humerus	Thoracodorsal (C6-C8)
Teres Major	Inferior angle of the scapula	Intertubercular groove of the humerus	Lower subscapular (C5-C6)
Subscapularis	Subscapular fossa	Lesser tuberosity of the humerus	Upper and lower subscapular (C5-C6)
Pectoralis Major	Sternal end of the clavicle and the sternocostal joints of ribs 1-7	Greater tubercle of the humerus	Medial (C8-T1) and lateral pectoral (C5-C7)

Glenohumeral Internal Rotation			
Muscle	**Origin**	**Insertion**	**Innervation**
Deltoid	Lateral third of the clavicle, acromion, and scapular spine	Deltoid tuberosity of the humerus	Axillary (C5-C6)
Infraspinatus	Infraspinous fossa	Greater tubercle of the humerus	Suprascapular (C4-C6)
Teres Minor	Lateral border of the scapula	Greater tuberosity of the humerus	Axillary (C5-C6)

FIG 3.52

Anatomy of the Third Cardinal Arm Movement: Considerations of Structures Affected

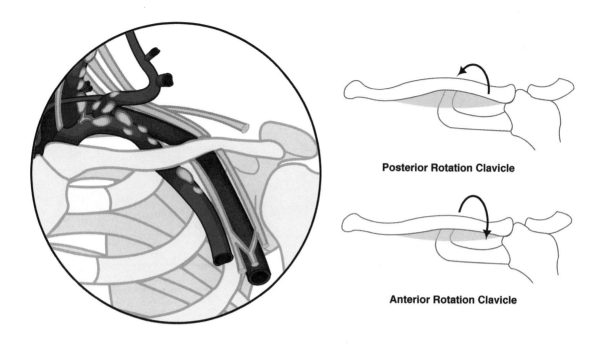

Posterior Rotation Clavicle

Anterior Rotation Clavicle

Rotation of the Clavicle

While balancing the upper T-Line on the transverse plane, the anterior and posterior rotation of the clavicle places compression on and off of the neurovascular structures between the first rib and the clavicle respectively.
This encourages the exchange of fluids within the upper extremity as well as drainage of the thoracic ducts.

Considerations of structures passing between the clavicle and 1st rib.

Brachial Plexus
Subclavian Artery + branches
Subclavian Vein + tributaries
Thoracic Ducts
Subclavian Lymph Trunks
Axillary Lymph Nodes
Pectoral Lymph Nodes

* The above chart demonstrates only a sampling of structures that may be affected.

FIG 3.53

Anatomy of the Cardinal Arm Movements: Brachial Plexus (Sites of potential obstruction)

Dorsal Scapular Nerve (C4-C5)

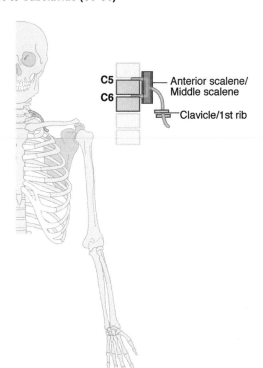

Suprascapular Nerve (C5-C6)

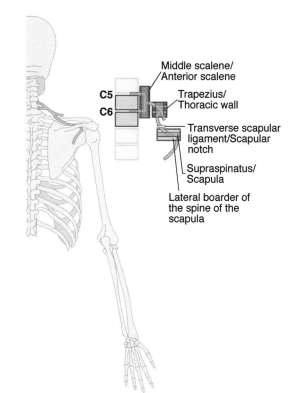

Nerve to Subclavius (C5-C6)

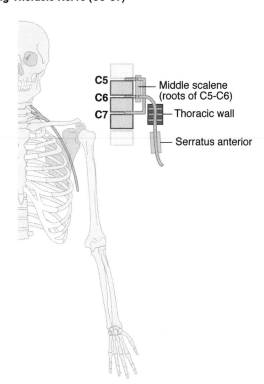

Long Thoracic Nerve (C5-C7)

FIG 3.54(a)

Subscapular Nerve (C5-C6)

Thoracodorsal Nerve (C6-C8)

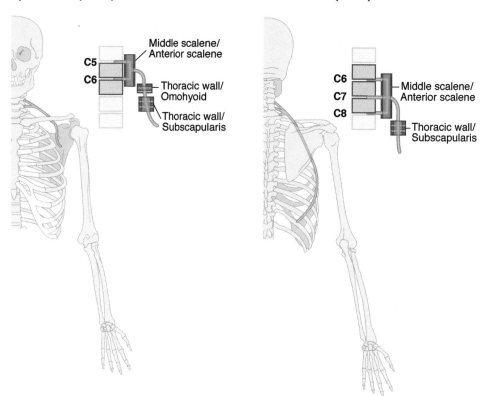

Subscapular Nerve labels:
- Middle scalene/Anterior scalene
- C5
- C6
- Thoracic wall/Omohyoid
- Thoracic wall/Subscapularis

Thoracodorsal Nerve labels:
- C6
- C7
- C8
- Middle scalene/Anterior scalene
- Thoracic wall/Subscapularis

Axillary Nerve (C5-C6)

Radial Nerve (C5-T1)

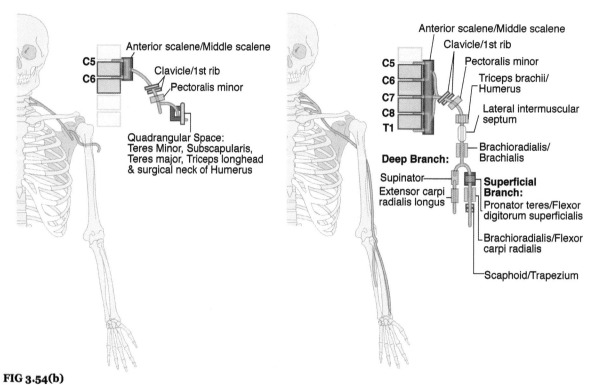

Axillary Nerve labels:
- C5
- C6
- Anterior scalene/Middle scalene
- Clavicle/1st rib
- Pectoralis minor
- Quadrangular Space: Teres Minor, Subscapularis, Teres major, Triceps longhead & surgical neck of Humerus

Radial Nerve labels:
- Anterior scalene/Middle scalene
- Clavicle/1st rib
- Pectoralis minor
- C5
- C6
- C7
- C8
- T1
- Triceps brachii/Humerus
- Lateral intermuscular septum
- Brachioradialis/Brachialis
- **Deep Branch:**
- Supinator
- Extensor carpi radialis longus
- **Superficial Branch:**
- Pronator teres/Flexor digitorum superficialis
- Brachioradialis/Flexor carpi radialis
- Scaphoid/Trapezium

FIG 3.54(b)

Medial + Lateral Pectoral Nerves (C5-T1)

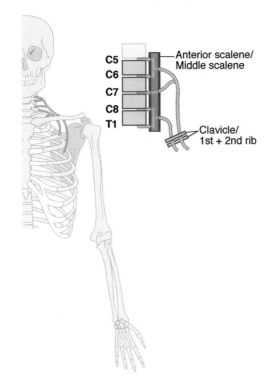

Musculocutaneous Nerve (C5-C7)

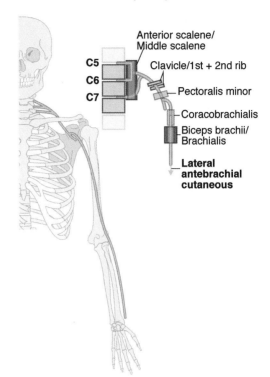

Ulnar Nerve (C8-T1)

Median Nerve (C6-T1)

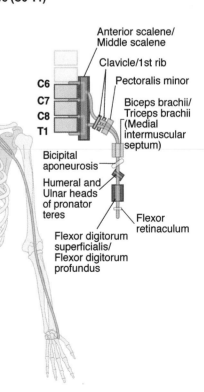

FIG 3.54(c)

Anatomy of the Cardinal Arm Movements: Arteries of the Thorax (Sites of potential obstruction)

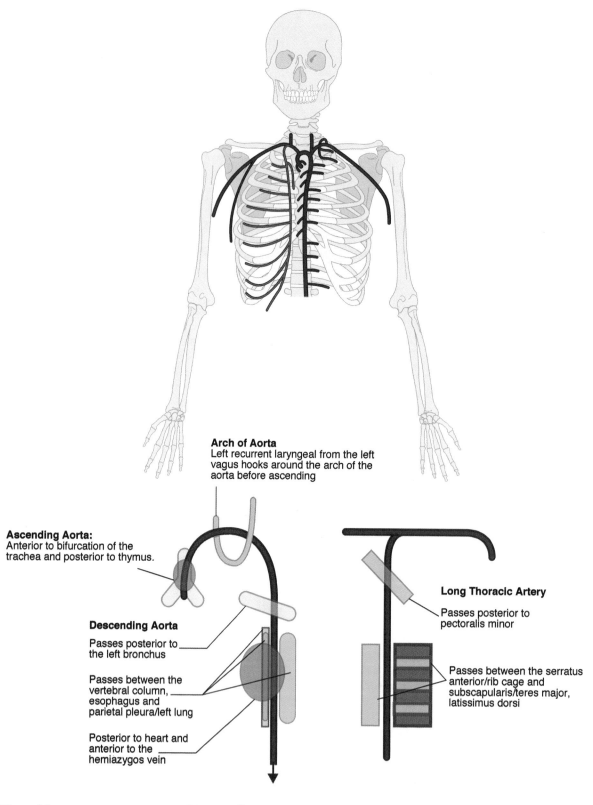

Arch of Aorta
Left recurrent laryngeal from the left vagus hooks around the arch of the aorta before ascending

Ascending Aorta:
Anterior to bifurcation of the trachea and posterior to thymus.

Descending Aorta

Passes posterior to the left bronchus

Passes between the vertebral column, esophagus and parietal pleura/left lung

Posterior to heart and anterior to the hemiazygos vein

Long Thoracic Artery

Passes posterior to pectoralis minor

Passes between the serratus anterior/rib cage and subscapularis/teres major, latissimus dorsi

FIG 3.55(a)

* Note: Not all arteries of the thorax are represented.

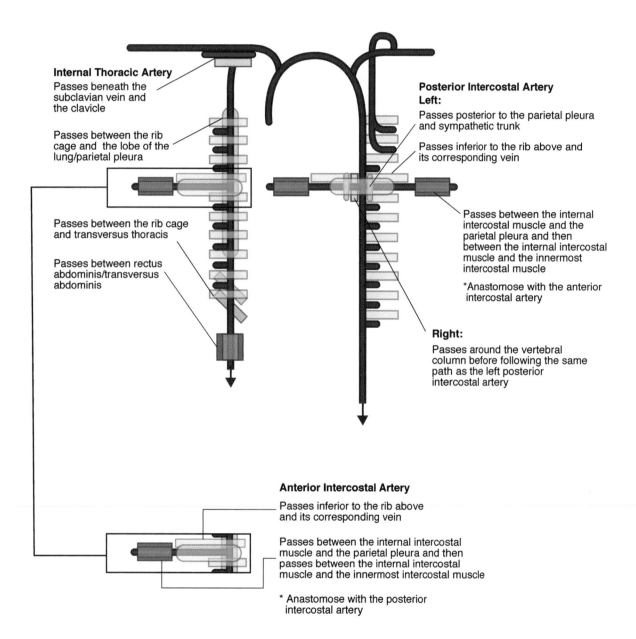

Internal Thoracic Artery

Passes beneath the
subclavian vein and
the clavicle

Passes between the rib
cage and the lobe of the
lung/parietal pleura

Passes between the rib cage
and transversus thoracis

Passes between rectus
abdominis/transversus
abdominis

Posterior Intercostal Artery
Left:

Passes posterior to the parietal pleura
and sympathetic trunk

Passes inferior to the rib above and
its corresponding vein

Passes between the internal
intercostal muscle and the
parietal pleura and then
between the internal intercostal
muscle and the innermost
intercostal muscle

*Anastomose with the anterior
 intercostal artery

Right:

Passes around the vertebral
column before following the same
path as the left posterior
intercostal artery

Anterior Intercostal Artery

Passes inferior to the rib above
and its corresponding vein

Passes between the internal intercostal
muscle and the parietal pleura and then
passes between the internal intercostal
muscle and the innermost intercostal muscle

* Anastomose with the posterior
  intercostal artery

FIG 3.55(b)   * Note: Not all arteries of the thorax are represented.

Anatomy of the Cardinal Arm Movements: Veins of the Thorax (Sites of potential obstruction)

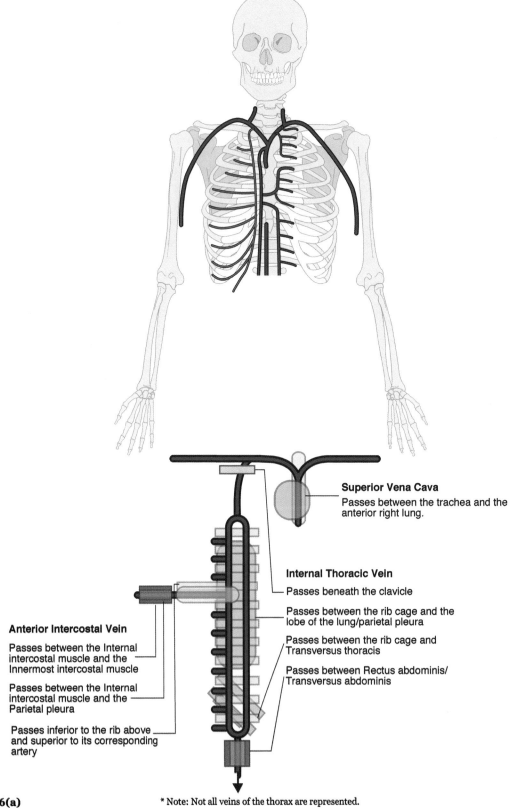

Superior Vena Cava

Passes between the trachea and the anterior right lung.

Internal Thoracic Vein

Passes beneath the clavicle

Passes between the rib cage and the lobe of the lung/parietal pleura

Passes between the rib cage and Transversus thoracis

Passes between Rectus abdominis/ Transversus abdominis

Anterior Intercostal Vein

Passes between the Internal intercostal muscle and the Innermost intercostal muscle

Passes between the Internal intercostal muscle and the Parietal pleura

Passes inferior to the rib above and superior to its corresponding artery

FIG 3.56(a)

* Note: Not all veins of the thorax are represented.

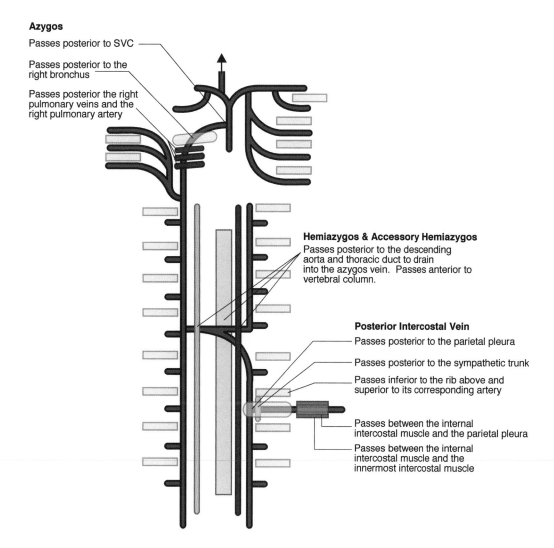

Azygos

Passes posterior to SVC

Passes posterior to the right bronchus

Passes posterior the right pulmonary veins and the right pulmonary artery

Hemiazygos & Accessory Hemiazygos
Passes posterior to the descending aorta and thoracic duct to drain into the azygos vein. Passes anterior to vertebral column.

Posterior Intercostal Vein

Passes posterior to the parietal pleura

Passes posterior to the sympathetic trunk

Passes inferior to the rib above and superior to its corresponding artery

Passes between the internal intercostal muscle and the parietal pleura

Passes between the internal intercostal muscle and the innermost intercostal muscle

FIG 3.56(b)   * Note: Not all veins of the thorax are represented.

Anatomy of the Cardinal Arm Movements: Arteries of the Upper Extremity (Sites of potential obstruction)

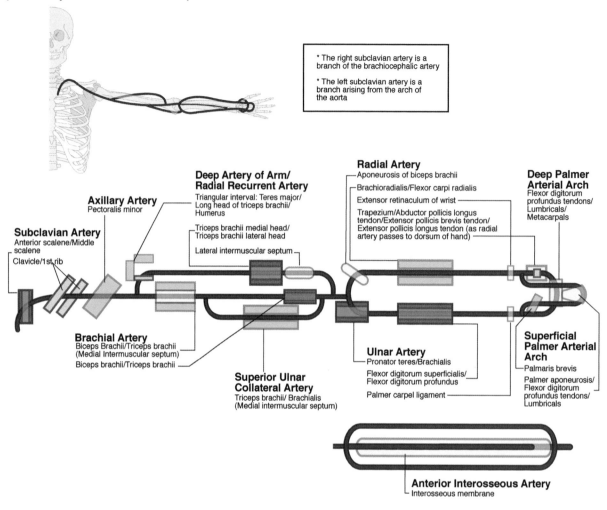

* The right subclavian artery is a branch of the brachiocephalic artery

* The left subclavian artery is a branch arising from the arch of the aorta

Subclavian Artery
Anterior scalene/Middle scalene
Clavicle/1st rib

Axillary Artery
Pectoralis minor

Deep Artery of Arm/ Radial Recurrent Artery
Triangular interval: Teres major/ Long head of triceps brachii/ Humerus
Triceps brachii medial head/ Triceps brachii lateral head
Lateral intermuscular septum

Radial Artery
Aponeurosis of biceps brachii
Brachioradialis/Flexor carpi radialis
Extensor retinaculum of wrist
Trapezium/Abductor pollicis longus tendon/Extensor pollicis brevis tendon/ Extensor pollicis longus tendon (as radial artery passes to dorsum of hand)

Deep Palmer Arterial Arch
Flexor digitorum profundus tendons/ Lumbricals/ Metacarpals

Brachial Artery
Biceps Brachii/Triceps brachii (Medial Intermuscular septum)
Biceps brachii/Triceps brachii

Superior Ulnar Collateral Artery
Triceps brachii/ Brachialis (Medial intermuscular septum)

Ulnar Artery
Pronator teres/Brachialis
Flexor digitorum superficialis/ Flexor digitorum profundus
Palmer carpel ligament

Superficial Palmer Arterial Arch
Palmaris brevis
Palmer aponeurosis/ Flexor digitorum profundus tendons/ Lumbricals

Anterior Interosseous Artery
Interosseous membrane

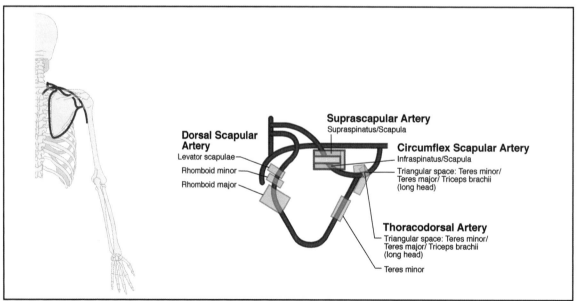

Dorsal Scapular Artery
Levator scapulae
Rhomboid minor
Rhomboid major

Suprascapular Artery
Supraspinatus/Scapula

Circumflex Scapular Artery
Infraspinatus/Scapula
Triangular space: Teres minor/ Teres major/ Triceps brachii (long head)

Thoracodorsal Artery
Triangular space: Teres minor/ Teres major/ Triceps brachii (long head)
Teres minor

FIG 3.57   * Note: Not all arteries of the upper extremity are represented.

Anatomy of the Cardinal Arm Movements: Veins of the Upper Extremity (Sites of potential obstruction)

Superficial Venous Drainage

Deep Venous Drainage

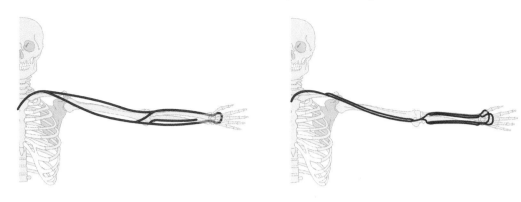

Superficial Venous Drainage

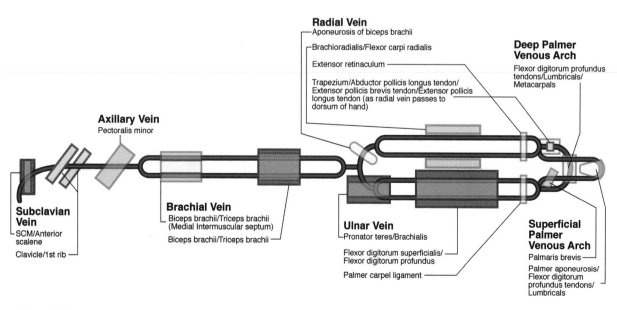

Cephalic Vein
Runs under the subcutaneous tissue and perforates the costocoracoid membrane and clavipectoral fascia

— Pectoralis major/Deltoid

Basilic Vein
Runs under the subcutaneous tissue and perforates the brachial fascia

— Pectoralis Major

Dorsal Venous network/ Median cubital Vein
Runs under the subcutaneous tissue

Deep Venous Drainage

Radial Vein
— Aponeurosis of biceps brachii

— Brachioradialis/Flexor carpi radialis

— Extensor retinaculum

— Trapezium/Abductor pollicis longus tendon/ Extensor pollicis brevis tendon/Extensor pollicis longus tendon (as radial vein passes to dorsum of hand)

Deep Palmer Venous Arch
Flexor digitorum profundus tendons/Lumbricals/ Metacarpals

Axillary Vein
Pectoralis minor

Subclavian Vein
└ SCM/Anterior scalene

Clavicle/1st rib ┘

Brachial Vein
└ Biceps brachii/Triceps brachii (Medial Intermuscular septum)

Biceps brachii/Triceps brachii ┘

Ulnar Vein
└ Pronator teres/Brachialis

Flexor digitorum superficialis/ Flexor digitorum profundus

Palmer carpel ligament

Superficial Palmer Venous Arch
Palmaris brevis ──

Palmer aponeurosis/ Flexor digitorum profundus tendons/ Lumbricals

FIG 3.58(a)

* Note: Not all veins of the upper extremity are represented.

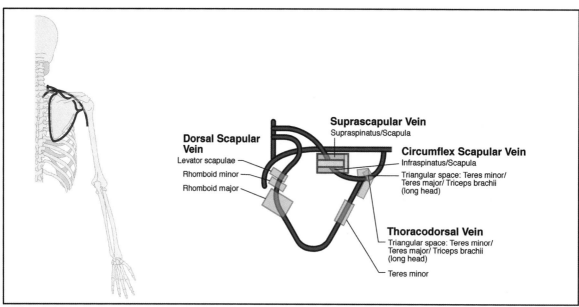

Dorsal Scapular Vein
Levator scapulae
Rhomboid minor
Rhomboid major

Suprascapular Vein
Supraspinatus/Scapula

Circumflex Scapular Vein
Infraspinatus/Scapula
Triangular space: Teres minor/
Teres major/ Triceps brachii
(long head)

Thoracodorsal Vein
Triangular space: Teres minor/
Teres major/ Triceps brachii
(long head)
Teres minor

FIG 3.58(b)

Anatomy of the Cardinal Arm Movements: Lymphatics of the Upper Extremity (Sites of potential obstruction)

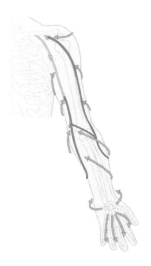

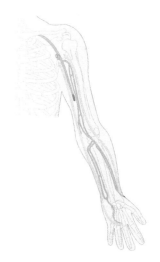

Superficial Lymphatic Drainage Upper Extremity

Superficial lymphatic drainage of the upper extremity begins in the skin of the hand and ascends along the paths of the superficial veins (Cephalic, Basilic).

Deep Lymphatic Drainage Upper Extremity

Deep lymphatic drainage of the upper extremity follows the deep veins (Radial, Ulnar and Brachial).

FIG 3.59(a)

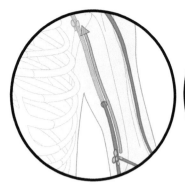

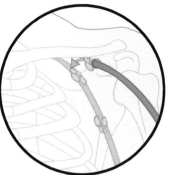

**Cubital Lymph Nodes to
Humeral Axillary Lymph Nodes**

**Deltopectoral Lymph Nodes to
Apical Axillary Lymph Nodes**

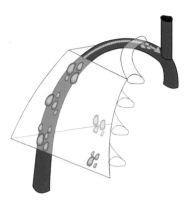

**Apical Axillary lymph nodes to
Lymphatic Duct via Subclavian trunk**

Path: Superficial Drainage of Upper Extremity

The lymph from the superficial upper extremity that drains along the basilic vein into the cubital lymph nodes, continues proximally to drain into the humeral axillary lymph nodes at the axilla. The superficial lymph following the basilic vein must pass through:

- Brachial fascia
- Pectoralis major

The lymph from the superficial upper extremity that drains along the cephalic vein will drain into the apical axillary lymph nodes. Some fluid may first pass through the deltopectoral lymph nodes. The superficial lymph following the cephalic vein must pass through:

- Pectoralis fascia
- Pectoralis major

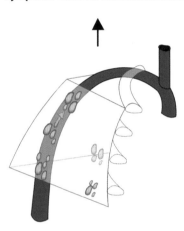

**Central Axillary lymph nodes to
Apical Axillary lymph nodes**

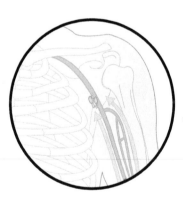

Path: Deep Drainage of Upper Extremity

The deep lymphatic drainage of the upper extremity follows the deep veins to drain into the humeral axillary lymph nodes. The deep veins pass through:

- Medial intermuscular septum (between biceps brachii and triceps brachii)
- Flexor compartment of antebrachium + Extensor retinaculum (ulnar vein)
- Bicipital aponeurosis + Extensor retinaculum (radial vein)

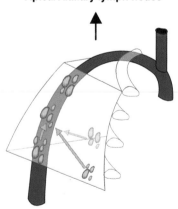

Path: Lymphatic Drainage of the Axilla
Lymphatic fluid, from both the superficial and deep lymph nodes, in the upper extremity drains through the axilla. The humeral axillary lymph nodes, the subscapular lymph nodes and the pectoral lymph nodes drain towards the central axillary lymph nodes.

FIG 3.59(b)

Anatomy of the Thorax: Lymphatic Drainage

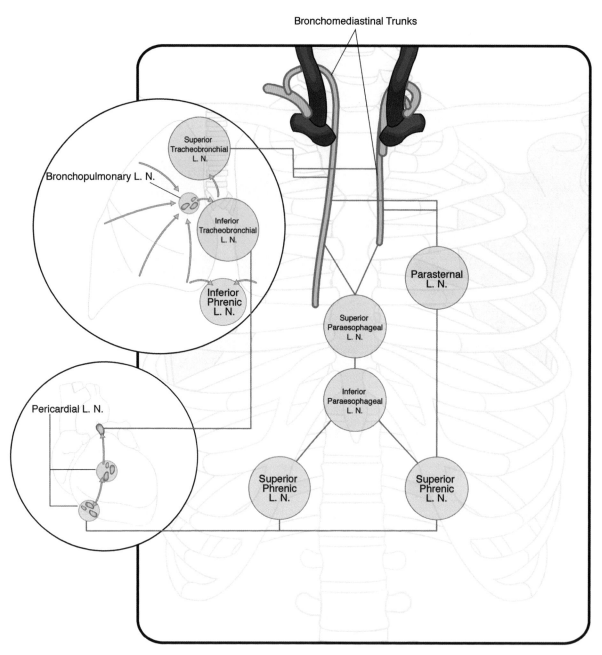

Thoracic Drainage via
Bronchomediastinal Trunks

Lymphatic Drainage of the Thorax

Drainage of the viscera and visceral pleura via:
- Bronchopulmonary lymph nodes to the tracheobronchial lymph nodes
- Paraesophageal lymph nodes
- Paracardial lymph nodes

* Visceral lymphatic drainage travels via lymph nodes to the bronchomediastinal trunks.

FIG 3.60(a)

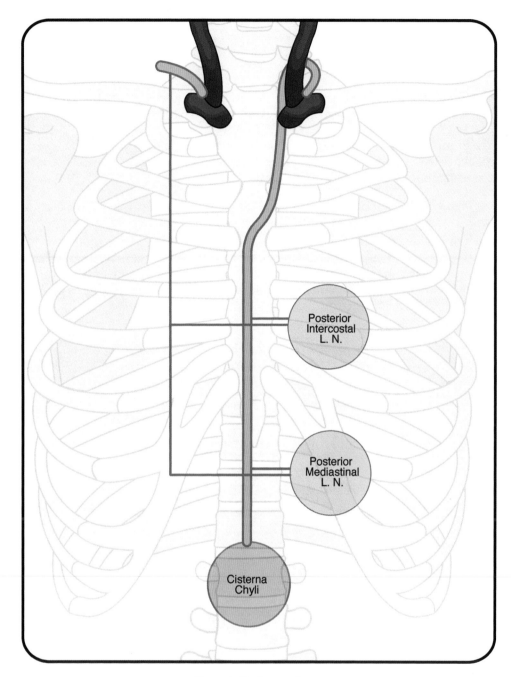

Thoracic Drainage via
Thoracic Duct/Right Lymphatic Duct

Lymphatic Drainage of the Thorax

Drainage of the thoracic wall and parietal Pleura via:
- Intercostal lymph nodes
- Parasternal lymph nodes
- Posterior mediastinal lymph nodes
- Diaphragmatic lymph nodes

* Superficial lymphatic drainage travels via lymph nodes to the thoracic duct or the bronchomediastinal trunks.

Superior Thoracic Aperture: Cervicothoracic Diaphragm

Addressing the superior thoracic aperture (STA) is also important for effective treatment, as the crucial neurovascular structures pass through it. The STA must especially be considered in treatments of the neck and cranium that involve drainage, and in treatments of the upper limb for neurovascular supply. The operator should be aware that restoring compliance to the aperture, which consists of the first thoracic vertebra, first two ribs, and manubrium, is the primary focus of the treatment.

The operator takes hold around the lateral aspect of the patient's neck such that his second digit rests at the sternoclavicular joint, and his third digit is below the clavicle at the connection of the first rib and sternum (**FIG. 3.61, 3.62**). Operators' third and fourth fingers splay over the chest wall and, depending on the size of the patient in relation to an operator's hands, their thumbs make contact with the posterior aspect of the patient's neck at a point just below the cervical column. This hold ensures that the operator has a flat hand on the bony ring that makes up the STA.

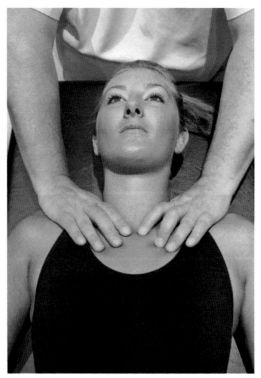 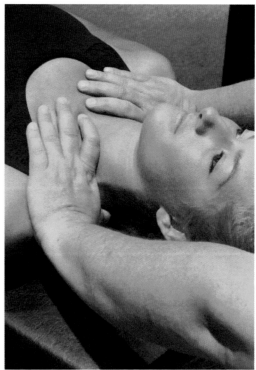

FIG 3.61 **FIG 3.62**

Hand position and body mechanics for treatment of the STA.

First, the operator can assess motion of the bony ring separately (yet in all planes) to ascertain the motion potential of the STA: flexion/extension in the sagittal plane, sidebending in the coronal plane, and rotation in the transverse plane (**FIG 3.63**). To induce movement in

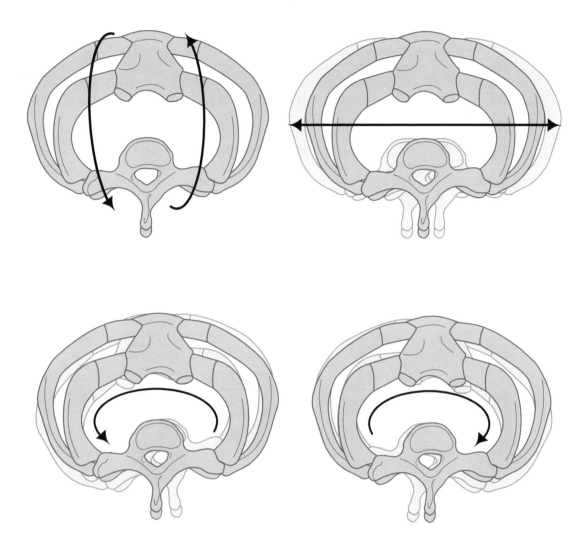

FIG 3.63: *Treating the superior thoracic aperture from the perspective of the operator.* Motion of the bony ring that makes up the superior thoracic aperture to treat the cervicothoracic diaphragm in the sagittal plane *(top, left)*, coronal plane *(top, right)*, and transverse plane *(bottom, left and right)* is illustrated. The darker portion of the image represents the neutral position of the STA which is superimposed over the lighter portion, representing the position of the STA after the motion is applied.

all of these planes, operators must have straight arms in order to transfer the motion from their body rather than inducing it via muscular strength (**FIG 3.64**).

For motion in the sagittal plane, the operator uses lean-on pressure to bring the STA into flexion—placing slight compression on the anterior aspect of the chest wall—and then leans off to bring it into extension. For motion in the coronal plane, the operator laterally transfers his hands from one side to the other, moving with his entire body. Lastly, for motion in the transverse plane, the operator can steer the patient into rotation by placing pressure through his palms towards the table. This last force is not directed downtable, but rather into the table to create rotation about a vertical axis. Directing force downtable would cause sidebending of the upper T-line in the coronal plane.

After operators have gained an understanding of the motion capacity of the patient's STA, they can apply treatment by stacking these planes. The first motion uses lean-on or lean-off pressure to facilitate motion within the sagittal plane until the operator reaches the barrier. Typically, either the patient's left or right side will have less range of motion than the other, and may require more pressure; thus, the operator's distribution of force may be unequal upon this first movement. While maintaining the barrier in the sagittal plane, the second motion is focused within the coronal plane. Here, just as they did in their assessment, operators transfer their hands and use their body to sidebend the STA. The operator brings the body just off midline to engage sidebending while maintaining their position in the sagittal plane. Depending on whichever side the operator moves, the STA there will be situated in a sidebending position in the opposite direction (**FIG 3.65, 3.66**). In other words, transferring the right hand toward the left hand will cause sidebending to the right, whereas transferring the left hand toward the right hand will cause sidebending to the left. The last motion is in the transverse plane to create rotation about a vertical axis. To do this—but without losing their position in the sagittal or coronal planes—operators should place pressure through their palm towards the table on the side in which they wish to induce rotation.

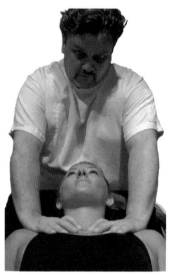
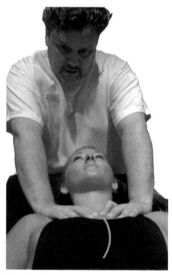
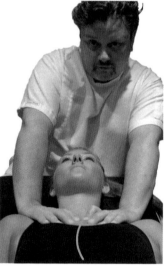

FIG 3.64: *Body mechanics during treatment of the STA.*

FIG 3.65

FIG 3.66

Body mechanics during sidebending of the STA. The STA undergoes sidebending to the side opposite that which operators move their hands, so that transferring to the left induces sidebending to the right and transferring to the right induces sidebending the left.

It is crucial to understand that motion in the sagittal plane will take up most of the available space, and that only fine tuning of the barrier will occur during sidebending and rotation of the STA. From here, the patient respires two to three times; this respiration helps the patient to engage their tissues in this new position, after which time the operator releases his hold upon the patient's inhalation. The operator can then motion test in a way similar to the methods used prior to treatment. The purpose of this test is to gauge whether the treatment effected a change.

Anatomy of the Superior Thoracic Aperture: Considerations of Structures Affected by Lesion

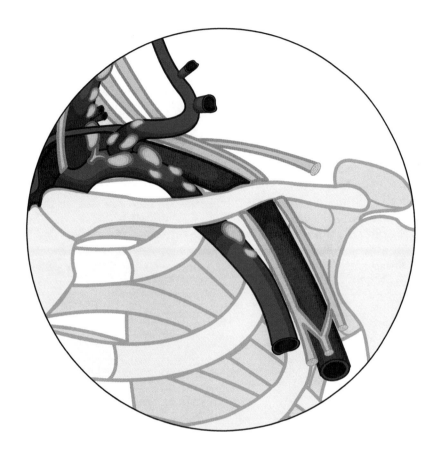

Considerations of structures that may be affected with a mechanical lesion of the STA.

Vagus Nerve (CNX)
Phrenic Nerve
Inferior Cervical Ganglion/Stellate Ganglion
Brachial Plexus
Brachiocephalic Trunk + branches
Subclavian Artery + branches
Internal Thoracic Artery
Brachiocephalic Vein + tributaries
Subclavian Vein + tributaries
Internal Thoracic Vein
Thoracic Ducts
Subclavian Lymph Trunks
Lungs
Endothoracic Fascia
Parietal and Visceral Pleura

* The above chart demonstrate only a sampling of
structures that may be affected.

FIG 3.67

Soft Tissue Preparation of the Cervical Spine

The cervical spine, similar to the lumbar spine, is an anterior curve, which means that the structural stability and integrity of the curve is largely maintained by the soft tissue that surrounds it. This is analogous to the way in which a string acts on a bow: an increase in the curvature of the bow (which in our case is the spine) will have a direct and proportional change to the tension in the string (or musculature), and vice versa (**FIG 3.68**). For this reason it is imperative to treat the soft tissue of the cervical spine before any diagnosis or treatment can be applied effectively to the hard tissue. The goal of this treatment is to address the soft tissue; thus, operators should be aware of their soft hold at the spine. If the patient's cervical spine is placed into extension, it is not merely unsafe for the patient. It also means that the operator has gone beyond the soft tissue articulation, and is instead at the hard tissue articulation. This is not the goal of this particular treatment. The following section will discuss preferred approaches to treating the tissues surrounding the cervical spine.

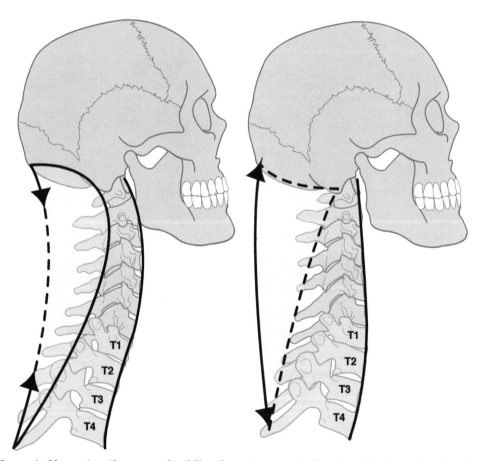

FIG 3.68: *The cervical bowstring.* The structural stability of anterior curves in the spine is largely attributed to the posterior soft tissue connected to them. As depicted in this image, an extension of the cervical spine leads to a more anteriorized curve, and thus to an approximation of the attachment points of this posterior musculature. Conversely, notice how flexion of the cervical spine leads to a more posteriorized curve and thus to more separational strain within the musculature.

Posterior Tissues

One approach to treating the entire musculature of the spinal column is through traction, the purpose of which is to increase spinal mobility by creating a separational strain between two attachment points of the soft tissue. As with any treatment, there are a variety of holds and approaches to traction that the operator can undertake (depending on the patient, of course), so long as each of those treatments adhere to the same principles. The following discussion will outline two holds that the operator can use to effect traction to the posterior tissues of the cervical spine.

Operators can overlap their hands, termed a *lap hold,* and support the cervical column such that the column itself lies on their fingers, and their thenar eminences act as an abutment at the occipitoatlantal sulcus (**FIG 3.69, 3.70**). Once the operator has a secure hold while maintaining soft and straight arms, he can simply lean back to create traction down the cervical spine. This hold is especially useful because there are multiple planes of motion available to the operator with little adjustment to the hand hold. Using their fingers, operators have the ability to easily add elements of flexion/extension, sidebending, and rotation to the cervical spine from the posterior aspect of the column (as necessary).

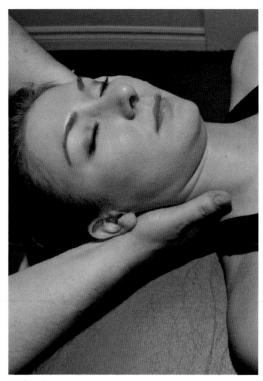
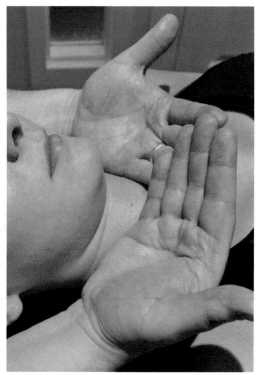

FIG 3.69

Lap hold of the cervical spine.

FIG 3.70

Another hold to create traction at the cervical spine involves the use of a *knife-edge* hold. Here, the operator uses slight adduction, or ulnar deviation, of one wrist. The wrist should be situated underneath the occipitoatlantal sulcus to support the head and neck. The operator can place his other hand either upon the patient's frontal bone with slight compression, or below the chin as a hook. Regardless of the hand position, both hands are used as a guide during traction. While dropping back with their body and straight arms, traction is applied to the cervical column using the sulcus as an abutment (employing the same method demonstrated above), but now with their knife-edge rather than their thenar eminences (**FIG 3.71, 3.72, 3.73**).

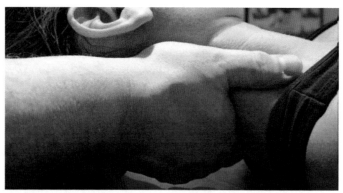

FIG 3.71

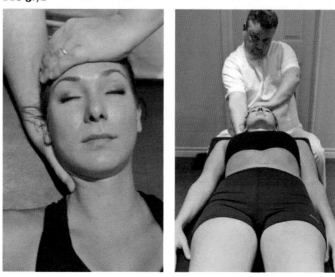

FIG 3.72   **FIG 3.73**

Knife-edge hold of the cervical spine and at the frontal bone.

Using either of these holds or any other that carries the same principles gives operators the ability to traction down to a desired level of the spine. They also have the ability to add an element of rotation to accompany the traction and articulate the tissues through coronal and transverse planes. To do this, operators maintain the traction through the lean-back shift of their body, but also shift their weight rhythmically from side to side. Since the functional movement of the cervical spine consists of sidebending and rotation correlated to the same side, there will be an element of sidebending accompanied with the rotation. While the operator moves to one side, he creates a traction down the opposite side of the cervical column (**FIG 3.74**). For example, the operator might shift his body weight to the appropriate target while tractioning down the left pillar of the cervical column. Operators may find that the patient prefers motion in one direction over the other; they can thus apply any approach to treat the barrier that is appropriate for the patient.

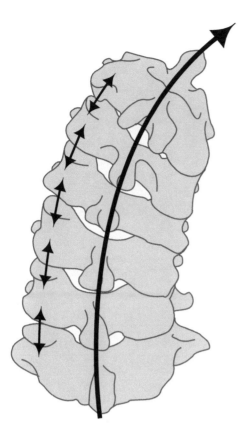

FIG 3.74: *Traction with accompanied articulation of the cervical spine.* While applying lean-back traction, the operator articulates the cervical spine by shifting his body weight to one side. In this example, while shifting to the right side of the body, the operator creates right sidebending and right rotation, motion mechanics that are dictated by the facet orientation of the lower cervical spine. This induces traction down the left pillar of the cervical column.

Operators can also choose to localize their traction to the cervical spine. To do this they can adjust their hand position such that one hand hold is more distal from them (closer to the thorax), and one is more proximal (closer to the cervical spine) (**FIG 3.75, 3.76**). A separational strain can then be created between these two points as the proximal hand drifts towards them away from the distal hand (**FIG 3.77**).

Aside from traction, the operator may also want to address the soft tissues by tractioning them lateralward from the nuchal ligament (**FIG 3.78**). Reaching across the table and behind the neck with his downtable hand, the operator grasps the posterior tissues with his finger pads (**FIG 3.79**). Operators may also wish to have their thenar eminence at the sternocleidomastoid (SCM) to incorporate it into the treatment (although another approach to treating this structure separately will be covered in more detail when we discuss treatment of the lateral tissues). The operator's uptable hand will direct the patient's head as a lever; the operator's hold will be at the frontal bone to facilitate rotation about a vertical axis. As they rotate the head towards their body, operators will guide the soft tissues along with the nuchal ligament laterally, yet in the opposite direction of the rotation. This is done to build posterior tension on the side opposite the rotation (**FIG 3.80**) and anterior at the SCM. As the head is rotated back to neutral, stopping before midline, the tissues come off of tension. By alternating between these rotations, the operator can approach the barrier to treat the posterior soft tissues.

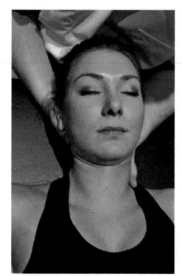 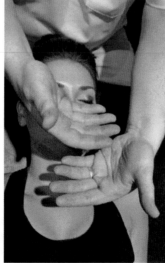 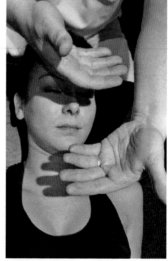

FIG 3.75   FIG 3.76   FIG 3.77

Separational strain created between two hands in the cervical spine.

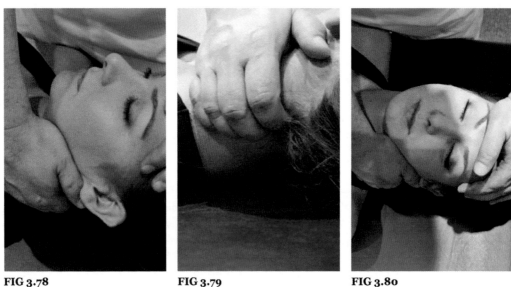

FIG 3.78   **FIG 3.79**   **FIG 3.80**

Addressing the soft tissues surrounding the nuchal ligament.

Lateral Tissues

The soft tissues that are of the utmost interest on the lateral aspect of the cervical spine include the SCM and the group of three scalenes. The purpose of the following discussion is to outline a variety of procedures the operator can apply to these important tissues. Of particular importance is the use of a soft but secure hold, as patient safety is of critical importance when working in the cervical spine area.

Treatment of the SCM is essential because it has a direct impact on the vagus and phrenic nerves as they travel toward the thorax. As discussed previously, this structure can be addressed in conjunction with the nuchal ligament—or separately—using a variety of different holds. The operator can use a positional approach to treatment by placing the head (which is, in essence, a long lever) in a position that isolates tension to the SCM, after which they may incorporate any myofascial treatment tool (**FIG 3.81, 3.82**). Alternatively, they may also choose to treat the structure using a short lever approach. Creating a *pincer grip*, the operator can use his hands as a wedge to traction the SCM off of the medial structures of the neck (**FIG 3.83, 3.84**). In the pincer grip, the SCM is isolated between the thumbs and forefingers, and the thenar eminences stabilize the hold against the lateral angle of the mandible.

The scalene muscles have a direct influence on the subclavian artery and vein, as well as on the brachial plexus, because these neurovascular structures weave between the muscles en route to the arm. Similar to the description above, where the operator uses the head to position the soft tissues to a point of tension, the operator can adjust the tissue in the scalenes by guiding the head into sidebending (**FIG 3.85**).

At this point the operator has a variety of tools to approach treatment of these lateral myofascial tissues. Should the operator wish to work in an indirect manner instead and bringing these tissues off tension, he would, of course, simply position the head in the opposite direction, and then proceed with treatment.

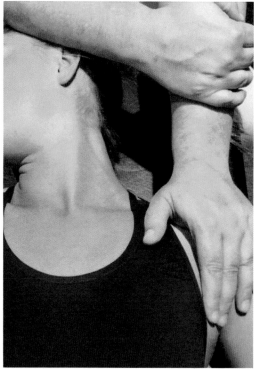
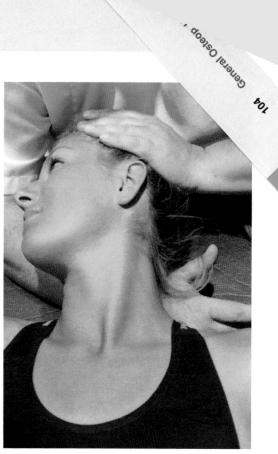

FIG 3.81

FIG 3.82

Long lever holds to generate tension on the sternocleidomastoid.

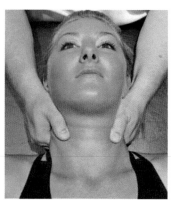
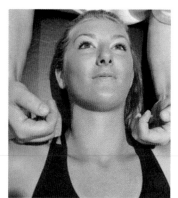
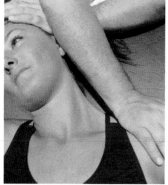

FIG 3.83

FIG 3.84

FIG 3.85: *Long lever hold to generate tension on the scalenes.*

Short lever hold to treat the sternocleidomastoid.

Anterior Tissues

Using the finger pads of their lateral digits, operators can carefully toggle the tissues of the anterior cervical spine right and left, and all the way up and down the anterior line from just below the oral diaphragm to the jugular notch at the manubrium. In this instance, operators utilize their fingers as a wedge to cause a shift in the tissues from midline, diagnosing and treating any asymmetries that may occur from side to side (**FIG 3.86, 3.87**).

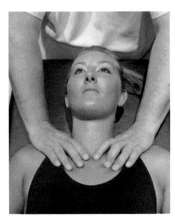 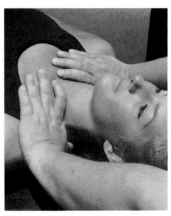

FIG 3.86   **FIG 3.87**

Treatment of structures on the anterior midline.

The transverse plane of musculature at the oral diaphragm is a key area to address to ensure there is proper drainage from the viscerocranium. The operator uses his finger pads to press along the inferior medial edge of the mandible at the oral diaphragm from the most anterior, midline portion, all the way to the most posterior and lateral aspect. At any point where they have diagnosed an asymmetry within this soft tissue, operators can move directly into treatment (**FIG 3.88, 3.89, 3.90**).

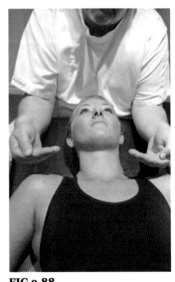 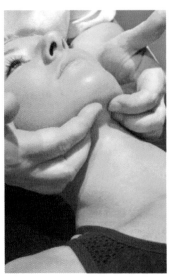 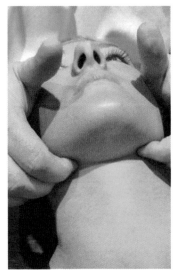

FIG 3.88   **FIG 3.89**   **FIG 3.90**

Treatment of the oral diaphragm.

Anatomy of the Neck: Cervical Plexus (Sites of potential obstruction)

Ansa Cervicalis Nerve (C1-C3)

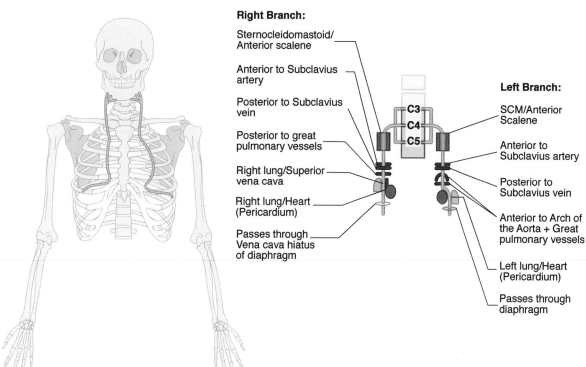

Superior Root:
Between the Internal jugular vein and Carotid artery
(within the Carotid sheath), beneath SCM

C1
C2
C3

Inferior Root:
SCM/Anterior scalene

Phrenic Nerve (C3-C5)

Right Branch:

Sternocleidomastoid/
Anterior scalene

Anterior to Subclavius
artery

Posterior to Subclavius
vein

Posterior to great
pulmonary vessels

Right lung/Superior
vena cava

Right lung/Heart
(Pericardium)

Passes through
Vena cava hiatus
of diaphragm

C3
C4
C5

Left Branch:

SCM/Anterior
Scalene

Anterior to
Subclavius artery

Posterior to
Subclavius vein

Anterior to Arch of
the Aorta + Great
pulmonary vessels

Left lung/Heart
(Pericardium)

Passes through
diaphragm

FIG 3.91(a)

Great Auricular Nerve (C2-C3)

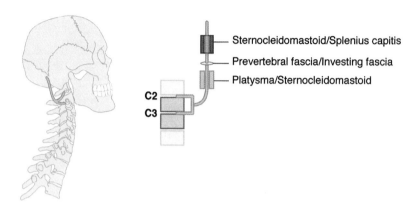

- Sternocleidomastoid/Splenius capitis
- Prevertebral fascia/Investing fascia
- Platysma/Sternocleidomastoid

C2
C3

Transverse Cervical Nerve (C2-C3)

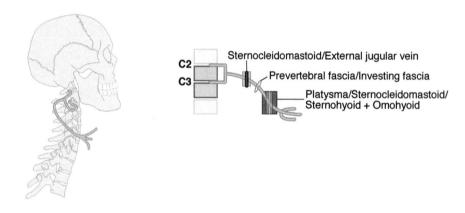

C2
C3

- Sternocleidomastoid/External jugular vein
- Prevertebral fascia/Investing fascia
- Platysma/Sternocleidomastoid/ Sternohyoid + Omohyoid

Lesser Occipital Nerve (C2-C3)

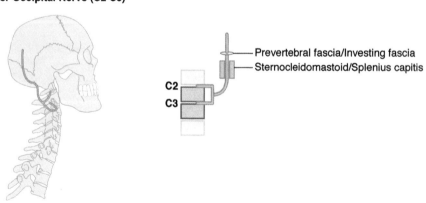

- Prevertebral fascia/Investing fascia
- Sternocleidomastoid/Splenius capitis

C2
C3

FIG 3.91(b)

Supraclavicular Nerves (C3-C4)

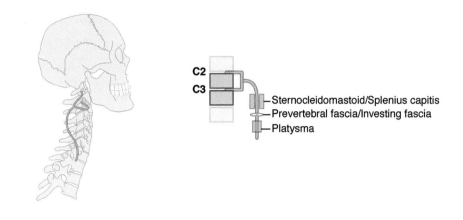

FIG 3.91(c)

Anatomy of the Neck: Considering the Sympathetic ANS

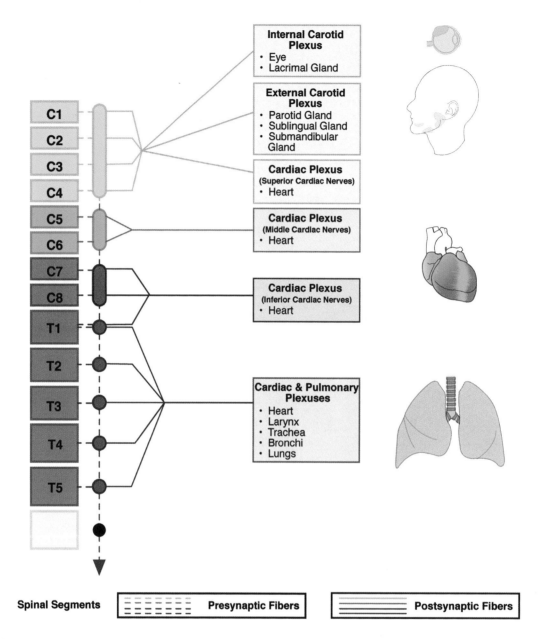

Considerations:

The inferior cervical ganglion (or stellate ganglion if combined with the first thoracic ganglion) is situated anterior to the neck of rib 1 and the TVP of C7. The middle cervical ganglion is located anterior to the TVPs of C5 and C6.

The superior cervical ganglion is located anterior to C1 and C2.

Thoracic sympathetic ganglia are located anterior to rib heads.

Therefore, mechanical lesions of the cervical vertebrae, ribs or STA may cause reflex effects via the ANS.

FIG 3.92

Anatomy of the Neck: Considering the Parasympathetic ANS

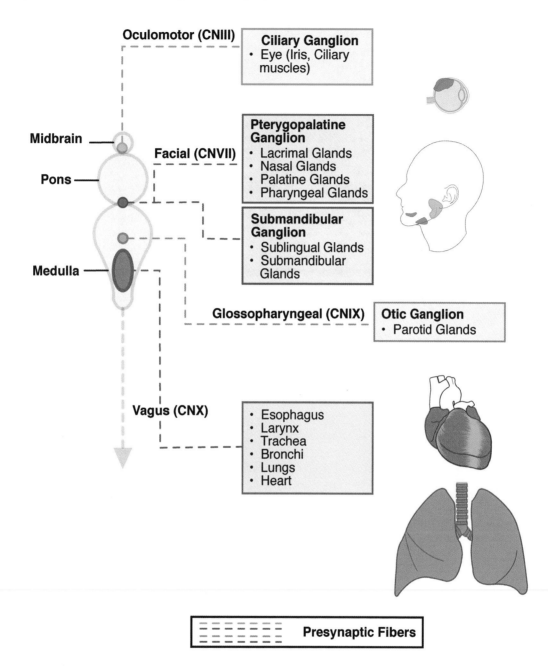

Ciliary Ganglion
• Eye (Iris, Ciliary muscles)

Oculomotor (CNIII)

Midbrain

Pons

Medulla

Pterygopalatine Ganglion
• Lacrimal Glands
• Nasal Glands
• Palatine Glands
• Pharyngeal Glands

Facial (CNVII)

Submandibular Ganglion
• Sublingual Glands
• Submandibular Glands

Glossopharyngeal (CNIX)

Otic Ganglion
• Parotid Glands

Vagus (CNX)

• Esophagus
• Larynx
• Trachea
• Bronchi
• Lungs
• Heart

▬ ▬ ▬ ▬ ▬ ▬ ▬ ▬   **Presynaptic Fibers**

Considerations:
The vagus nerve (CNX) is the principle nerve supplying parasympathetic innervation to the cardiopulmonary and digestive viscera. It may be disrupted by mechanical lesions at the cervical spine. See FIG 5.7 for the course of the vagus nerve

FIG 3.93

Anatomy of the Neck: Arteries (Sites of potential obstruction)

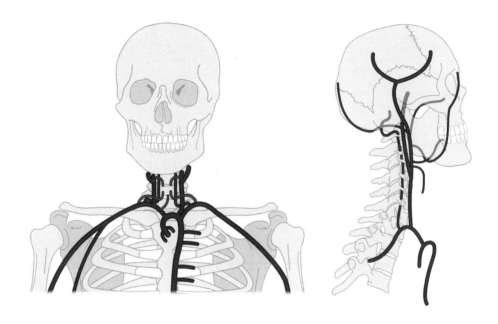

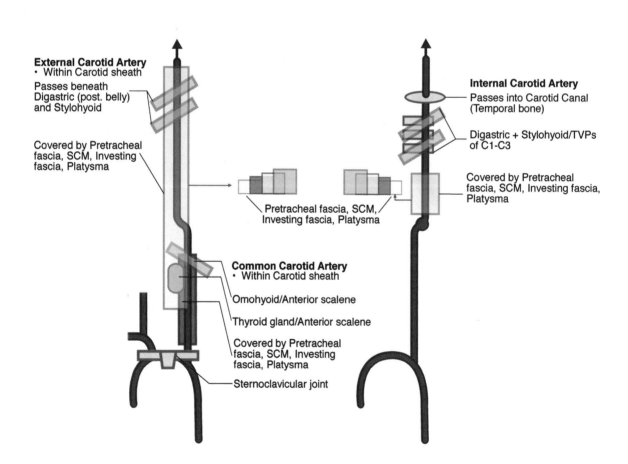

External Carotid Artery
- Within Carotid sheath

Passes beneath Digastric (post. belly) and Stylohyoid

Covered by Pretracheal fascia, SCM, Investing fascia, Platysma

Pretracheal fascia, SCM, Investing fascia, Platysma

Internal Carotid Artery

Passes into Carotid Canal (Temporal bone)

Digastric + Stylohyoid/TVPs of C1-C3

Covered by Pretracheal fascia, SCM, Investing fascia, Platysma

Common Carotid Artery
- Within Carotid sheath

Omohyoid/Anterior scalene

Thyroid gland/Anterior scalene

Covered by Pretracheal fascia, SCM, Investing fascia, Platysma

Sternoclavicular joint

FIG 3.94(a)

* Note: Not all arteries of the neck are represented.

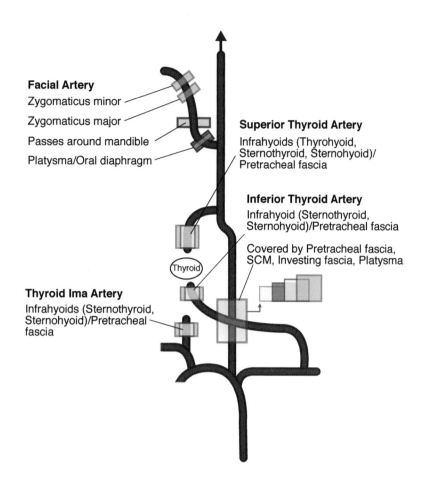

Facial Artery

Zygomaticus minor

Zygomaticus major

Passes around mandible

Platysma/Oral diaphragm

Superior Thyroid Artery

Infrahyoids (Thyrohyoid,
Sternothyroid, Sternohyoid)/
Pretracheal fascia

Inferior Thyroid Artery

Infrahyoid (Sternothyroid,
Sternohyoid)/Pretracheal fascia

Covered by Pretracheal fascia,
SCM, Investing fascia, Platysma

Thyroid

Thyroid Ima Artery

Infrahyoids (Sternothyroid,
Sternohyoid)/Pretracheal
fascia

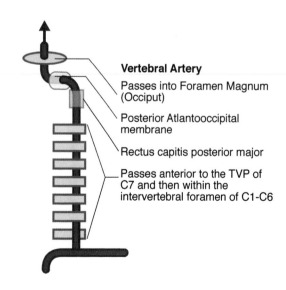

Vertebral Artery

Passes into Foramen Magnum
(Occiput)

Posterior Atlantooccipital
membrane

Rectus capitis posterior major

Passes anterior to the TVP of
C7 and then within the
intervertebral foramen of C1-C6

FIG 3.94(b)

Anatomy of the Neck: Veins (Sites of potential obstruction)

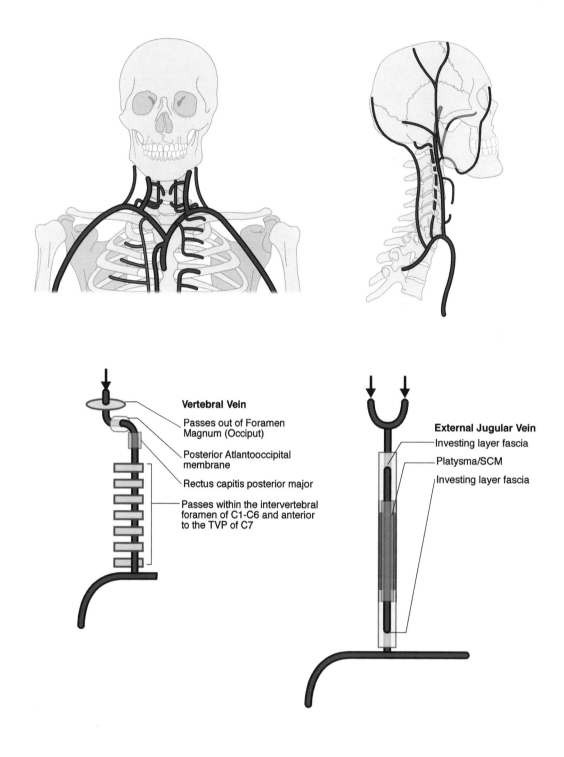

Vertebral Vein

Passes out of Foramen
Magnum (Occiput)

Posterior Atlantooccipital
membrane

Rectus capitis posterior major

Passes within the intervertebral
foramen of C1-C6 and anterior
to the TVP of C7

External Jugular Vein

Investing layer fascia

Platysma/SCM

Investing layer fascia

FIG 3.95(a)   * Note: Not all veins of the neck are represented.

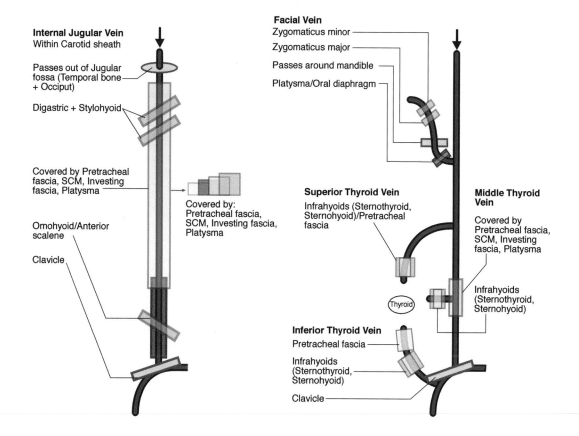

Internal Jugular Vein
Within Carotid sheath

Passes out of Jugular fossa (Temporal bone + Occiput)

Digastric + Stylohyoid

Covered by Pretracheal fascia, SCM, Investing fascia, Platysma

Covered by:
Pretracheal fascia, SCM, Investing fascia, Platysma

Omohyoid/Anterior scalene

Clavicle

Facial Vein
Zygomaticus minor
Zygomaticus major
Passes around mandible
Platysma/Oral diaphragm

Superior Thyroid Vein
Infrahyoids (Sternothyroid, Sternohyoid)/Pretracheal fascia

Middle Thyroid Vein
Covered by Pretracheal fascia, SCM, Investing fascia, Platysma

Infrahyoids (Sternothyroid, Sternohyoid)

Thyroid

Inferior Thyroid Vein
Pretracheal fascia

Infrahyoids (Sternothyroid, Sternohyoid)

Clavicle

FIG 3.95(b)   * Note: Not all veins of the neck are represented.

Anatomy of the Neck: Lymphatic Drainage

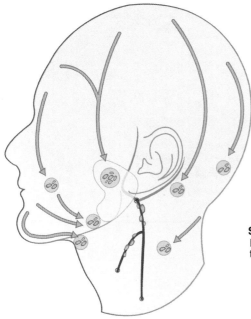

Superficial Lymph Nodes Head and Neck
Passes through the investing fascia to drain into the deep Cervical lymph nodes.

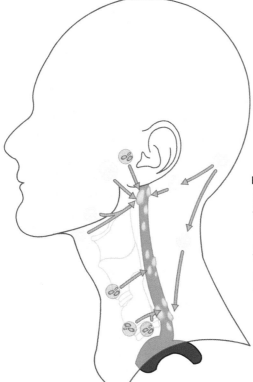

Deep Lymph Nodes Head and Neck
Deep cervical lymph nodes surrounding the internal jugular vein receive efferent lymph fluid from superficial and deep lymphatic glands.

Drainage of the deep cervical lymph nodes must pass under the sternocleidomastoid and the pretracheal fascia.

Drainage into the thoracic ducts may be affected by the articulation of the clavicle and sternum.

FIG 3.96(a)

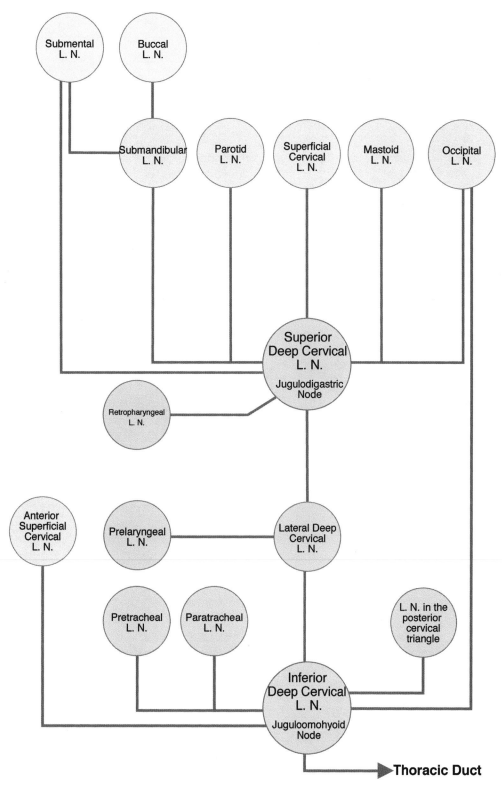

FIG 3.96(b)

Cranial Drainage

An important principle that governs the sequencing within treatment has to do with drainage and supply. In order to have the exchange of fluids within an area, there must be space into which the fluid can flow. Providing this space assists in creating a pressure gradient that draws fresh fluid into the newly created space. In other words, *drainage must precede supply*. When treating the cranium, the operator works within this principle by treating from the base upwards, creating space in the thorax into which fluid from the head and neck can drain. The succeeding treatment then addresses the head, neck, and face. The image below offers an example of a general drainage treatment for the face and cranium in the event of vascular congestion in the area. Over the course of this treatment, the operator will apply pressure to the crucial vascular routes that course through the viscerocranium in order to encourage the movement of fluids.

Beginning with their thumbs on the medial aspect of the frontal bone (**FIG 3.97**), the operator traces around the lateral aspect of the orbits, then traces medially across the zygomatic arch back towards the nose before coming back laterally around the angle of the jaw (**FIG 3.98**). At this point, operators can switch their handling from their thumb pad to their finger pads and follow along the lateral neckline near the SCM (**FIG 3.99**). This motion brings fluid from the face through the neck to drain back into central circulation, and is generally repeated as many times as necessary to clear any vascular congestion.

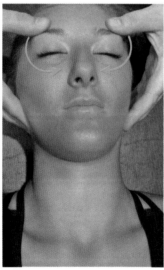 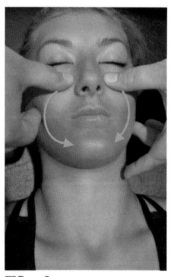 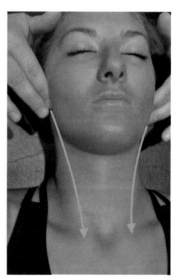

FIG 3.97   **FIG 3.98**   **FIG 3.99**

Vascular drainage of the viscerocranium.

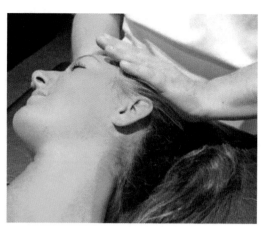

FIG 3.100: *Stimulation of the scalp.*

Now that the operator has helped to promote fluid drainage in the face, he can stimulate the scalp at various areas, shown here at the parietal eminence, to promote vasodilation in the cranium and thus the exchange of vascular fluid from deep to superficial (**FIG 3.100**).

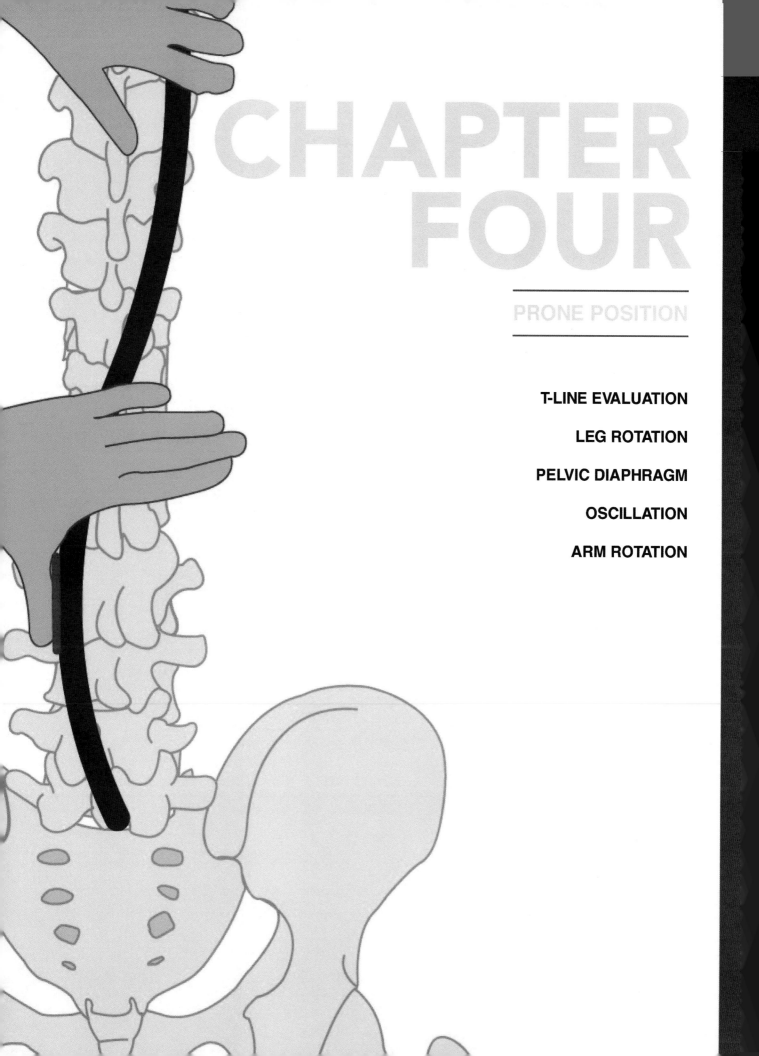

CHAPTER FOUR

PRONE POSITION

Lower T-Line Evaluation Using Long Levers: Telescoping

Similar to telescoping during the T-line evaluation while supine (described above), the lower T-line can be assessed in prone position using a bilateral or unilateral traction or compression by treating the legs as long levers. To assess the lower limbs or lower T-line bilaterally in this position, the operator cups the dorsal aspect of the foot and either drops backwards to apply traction, or leans forward to compress the chain (**FIG 4.1, 4.2**). A loss of pliability during this motion could indicate a lesion in the lower limb, or a declination/inclination in the lower T-line. This procedure can also be used to assess flexion and extension past the lower T-line and into the lumbars for movement in the sagittal plane. Operators can rest the patient's foot unilaterally on their hip and compress uptable, or use the hip as an abutment as they traction the other leg downtable (**FIG 4.3**). In this case, because the force is being transmitted unilaterally, the operator is no longer assessing flexion and extension but rather sidebending and rotation in the coronal and transverse planes, respectively.

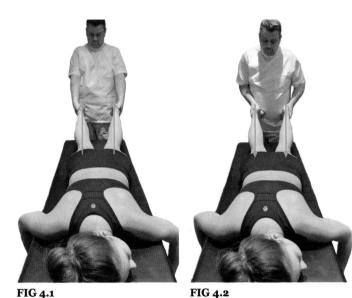
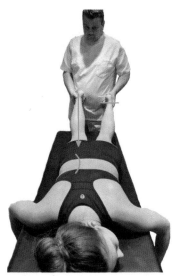

FIG 4.1   **FIG 4.2**

Bilateral assessment of the lower T-line using long levers in prone position with caudad traction and cephalad compression.

FIG 4.3: *Unilateral assessment of the lower T-line using long levers in prone position.*

Leg Rotation

Just as a supine leg rotation can be used to treat any joint up the chain of the lower limb and into the lower polygon, so too can a prone leg rotation be employed. An advantage to leg rotation in prone, as opposed to supine, is the freedom of motion directed to the sacrum, which makes it more effective to adjust in this position.

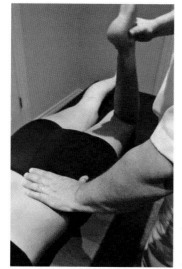

FIG 4.4: *Palpation of the sacroiliac and coxofemoral joints during prone leg rotation.*

Assessment begins as soon as the operator cups the foot at the dorsal aspect and brings the leg into flexion at the knee. The operator can assess the quality of motion at the coxofemoral joint by easily palpating motion at the greater trochanter (**FIG 4.4**). Frequently there will be a restriction at the femoral head and, consequently, this lesion must be addressed before moving more distally from the lever. As explained in a supine leg rotation, the leverage from the leg will not reach into the innominate if this joint is dysfunctional and unable to transmit the force. For example, if there is a lesion causing dysfunction in the lateral rotators, the operator may need to address the soft tissue before moving on past the hip in order to ensure the lever is functional. Staying within the sagittal plane, the further the operator brings the knee into flexion, the more tension he will induce on the ventral line of the lower limb. This tension could be used to treat an innominate lesion, for example, that may be inhibiting the transfer of force through the innominate and into the sacrum.

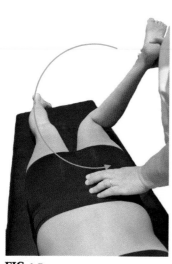

FIG 4.5

Prone leg rotation.

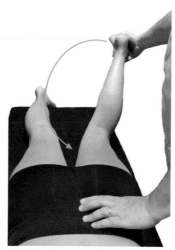

FIG 4.6

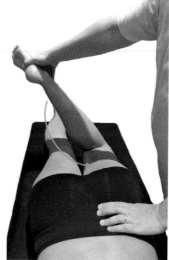

FIG 4.7

Once the operator has addressed the coxofemoral joint and innominates, thereby ensuring that the leg is a viable lever, he can now move more distally to these points. As the ankle is brought over the midline, the operator is inducing external rotation of the femoral head within the acetabulum, whereas bringing the ankle laterally induces internal rotation (**FIG 4.5, 4.6, 4.7**). If the operator has engaged the ligaments correctly, this external and internal rotation of the hip will enable a palpable closing/opening of the sacroiliac joint via out-flaring/inflaring the innominate, respectively. Through the anatomical connections of the lower limb the operator can use the leg as a long lever to treat the joints from the hip to the sacrum and lumbar spine, all while approaching the barrier model according to the lesion the patient presents.

Pelvic Diaphragm

After addressing the respiratory, cervicothoracic, and oral diaphragm in supine position, the last diaphragm to be discussed will be those muscles that make up the pelvic diaphragm. It is an important group of soft tissues to address, especially when working with the sacrum.

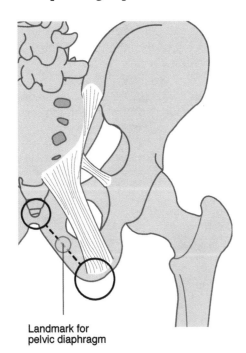

Landmark for
pelvic diaphragm

FIG 4.8: *Landmarking the pelvic diaphragm.*

To landmark the pelvic diaphragm, operators use their uptable hand to locate the coccyx and their downtable hand to landmark the ischial tuberosity (**FIG 4.8, 4.9**). Drawing a diagonal line between these two points, which roughly represents the fibres of the sacrotuberous ligament, the operator can use both thumbs to mark the middle of this line (**FIG 4.10**). With a thumb-over-thumb hold, operators can grasp the gluteal tissues with their fingers to slacken the soft tissue at their thumbs (**FIG 4.11**), and then sink in on a nearly vertical direction toward the table. Curling their thumbs laterally into the soft tissue barrier, operators should be beneath the ligamentous structures and reach the pelvic diaphragm (**FIG 4.12, 4.13**). As the patient respires, the operator should feel the diaphragm descend upon inhalation and ascend upon exhalation. By following similar principles as those used for the treatment of the respiratory diaphragm, the operator already has an approach to directly treat the soft tissues of the pelvic floor.

The operator, however, should keep in mind the mechanical and neurophysiological aspects of the pelvic floor (such as the bony attachments and neural input), and incorporate these structures into treatment to fully stabilize the lumbopelvic area.

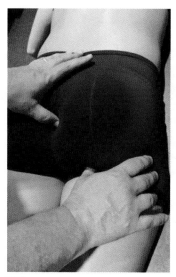 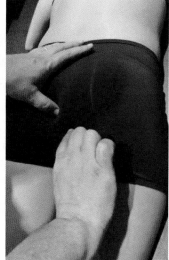 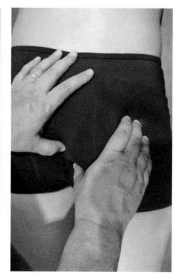

FIG 4.9   FIG 4.10   FIG 4.11

Landmarking the pelvic diaphragm.

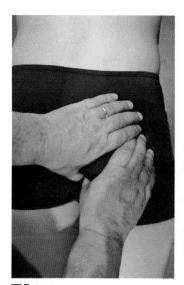 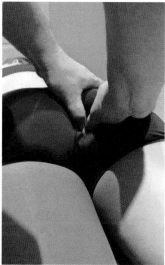

FIG 4.12   FIG 4.13

Sinking into the soft tissues of the pelvic diaphragm.

Anatomy of the Pelvic Diaphragm: Related Fascia

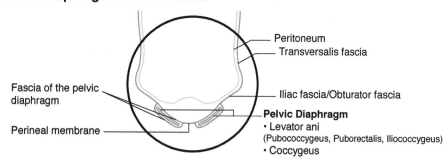

Peritoneum
Transversalis fascia

Fascia of the pelvic
diaphragm

Iliac fascia/Obturator fascia

Pelvic Diaphragm
• Levator ani
(Pubococcygeus, Puborectalis, Iliococcygeus)
• Coccygeus

Perineal membrane

FIG 4.14

Oscillation

Oscillation is a tool that the operator can use to find or initiate the rhythm that complements the natural rhythm of the patient's body. It can be used as a tool to integrate structures and their movements, as a tool to calm the patient (as it is soothing to the nervous system), or in combination with a fulcrum treatment to direct movement to a specific point in the soft or hard tissues. In the latter case, this technique improves the articulation, or congruency, between soft and hard tissue surfaces. Oscillation can even be used as a tool to move fluids—once diaphragms have been addressed—by increasing the speed of the oscillation. The operator can move easily in and out of diagnosis and treatment when oscillating, as it provides an impression of the motion available at a desired point in all planes. Once the operator has made a diagnosis, he can move on and off the barrier as necessary to induce motion up to, or at the point of, the fulcrum. In this example, oscillation beginning at the sacrum will illustrate how movement can be induced, transferred, and used as a tool to treat the spinal column.

The operator stands close to the table and, with straight arms, places his thenar eminence softly on the lateral aspect of the sacrum nearest to him. Using a steady, rhythmic pulse, the operator creates a rocking motion from his body that transfers through the arm and hands to the sacrum (**FIG 4.15, 4.16**). Because of the location of the hand, a separational strain is induced between the sacrum and the innominate at the sacroiliac joint.

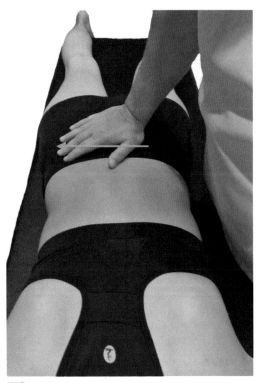 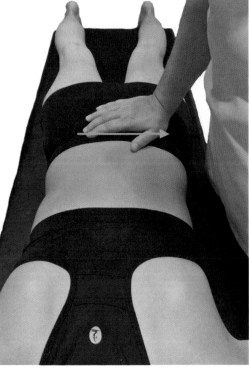

FIG 4.15
Oscillation of the sacrum.

FIG 4.16

Once the operator has a steady rhythm, the initial movements are diagnostic, as he can assess how the motion moves through the body. It is imperative that the operator has the patient set up properly in order for this oscillation to carry through the body; for example, in cases of lordosis, the operator should pillow the lumbars so that the spine is brought into a neutral position and motion is not altered by the articulation of the spinal facets upon one another. Such an articulation would create new pivot points for the induced motion. Similarly, the patient's feet should be situated just off of the table so that the patient's toes do not stop the oscillation through the lower limbs, and so that there is no anterior or posterior tension travelling through the soft tissue of the lower limbs.

As the oscillation travels through the body, operators can use their uptable hand to assess motion at the spine. Using a straight thumb to create a vertical line, they can rest this on the lateral aspect most proximal to them, but spanning two or three spinous processes (**FIG 4.17**). Similarly, operators can change their hand positioning such that they are using their fingertips on the lateral aspect most distal to them, again spanning two or three spinous processes but on the opposite side (**FIG 4.18**). Motion palpated using either of these holds can indicate a concavity or convexity over a local area when the movement of these vertebrae are compared to one another. Alternatively, a pincer grip on one segment provides more of a focal assessment that can be useful if we wish to assess or treat one vertebra in isolation. It does not, however, give us as much room to simultaneously compare the motion of one vertebra to another. Each hold of the spine that operators use must be carefully selected to match their intent, as different holds will each have their advantages and disadvantages.

In areas where operators palpate an asymmetry, they can create a fixed point upon which they focus their oscillation. They can also create a push with their thumb or pull with their fingertips to induce the convexity or concavity into or away from the barrier, depending on which tool is appropriate for that patient.

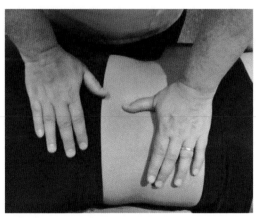 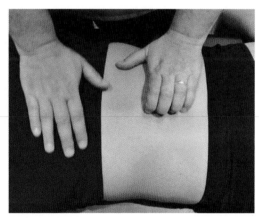

FIG 4.17   **FIG 4.18**

Using the uptable hand to push or pull the spine and create movement to a fixed point during oscillation.

Oscillation Review

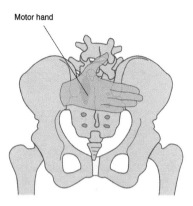

Motor hand

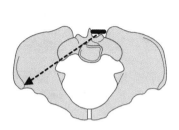

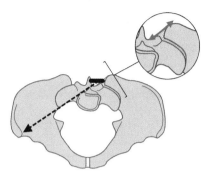

Landmarking
Place the thenar eminence on the lateral aspect of the sacrum. There is full hand contact.

Direction of Force
Using a steady, rhythmic pulse, the operator creates a rocking motion from his body that transfers through the arm and hand to the sacrum. The force is applied towards the ASIS on the contralateral side.

Effect
A separational strain is induced between the sacrum and the innominate at the sacroiliac joint.

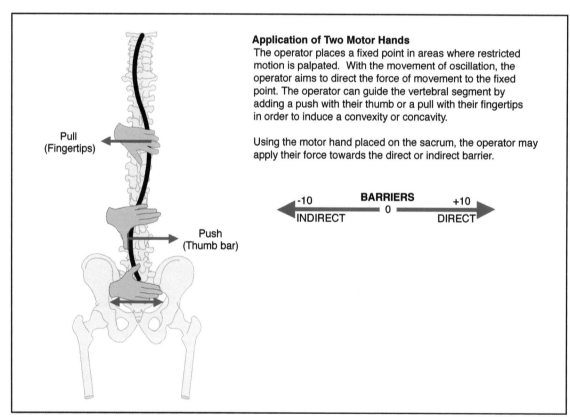

Pull
(Fingertips)

Push
(Thumb bar)

Application of Two Motor Hands
The operator places a fixed point in areas where restricted motion is palpated. With the movement of oscillation, the operator aims to direct the force of movement to the fixed point. The operator can guide the vertebral segment by adding a push with their thumb or a pull with their fingertips in order to induce a convexity or concavity.

Using the motor hand placed on the sacrum, the operator may apply their force towards the direct or indirect barrier.

BARRIERS

-10   0   +10

INDIRECT   DIRECT

FIG 4.19

Arm Rotation

The operator can utilize the shoulder girdle in prone to address the upper T-line. By nature of the anatomical arrangement of the shoulder joint, the operator can better assess and treat the soft tissue of the scapulothoracic joint (which has more freedom of motion in prone), as well as the lateral line of the upper polygon, the ventral line of the pectorals, and osseous articulations that contribute to the upper T-line.

Facing uptable in a fencer stance, the operator glides his uptable arm underneath the patient's own arm, and hooks into the cubital fossa so that the antebrachium supports the patient's brachium. The operator can cup the anterior portion of the glenohumeral joint, then stand to bring the shoulder girdle posterior. At this point operators should take note of their own body mechanics, ensuring that their posture is straight, and that any forward flexion they may need comes from their hips rather than their lumbar spine (**FIG 4.20**).

Using their body to induce motion, operators can bring the patient's shoulder girdle through rotation. With the patient lying on her ventral surface, the table acts as a fixed point on the sternal and costal attachment of the pectoralis muscle—which is the lateral line of the upper polygon—as the operator posteriorizes the shoulder girdle (**FIG 4.21**). Furthermore, the operator can use this lever to investigate the glenohumeral or scapulothoracic joints and, if the lever is functional, this arm revolution can be used to induce rotation in the spi-

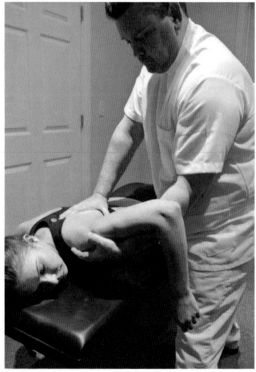

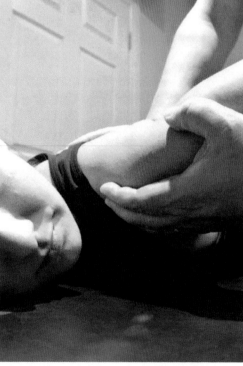

FIG 4.20: *Body mechanics during a prone arm rotation.*

FIG 4.21: *Hand positioning for a prone arm rotation.*

nal region around the mid-dorsals. Depending on the operator's intended function of the lever, he will use his downtable hand to palpate or create a fixed point in that area.

Because of the anatomical correlation from the shoulder girdle to the head, neck, and upper dorsals (through the soft tissue of the neck), it is necessary to discuss the position of the patient's head during this motion. Ideally, if the patient is capable of doing so, she should have her head rotated to the side on which the operator is working. This is advised in order to follow the rotation of the upper T-line induced by this motion.

At this point, an opportunity presents itself for the operator: that is, to compare his findings of this region to those in supine, and utilize the position accordingly. For example, if the operator wanted to treat a posterior shoulder issue diagnosed in supine using an indirect approach, it may be more advantageous to apply treatment in the prone position where the table does not block the operator's movement. This example offers the reader a glimpse into staging from one position to the next over the course of one treatment in order to make it safer, efficient, and effective.

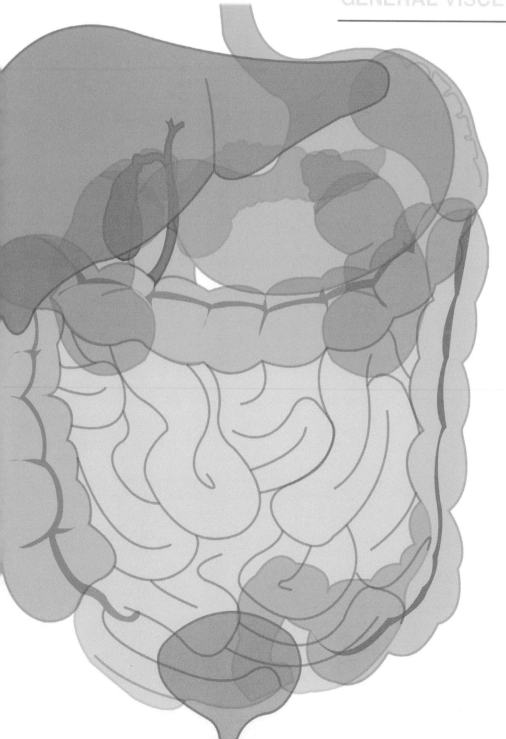

CHAPTER FIVE

GENERAL VISCERAL TREATMENT

...odominal Viscera Treatment: An Introduction

...ce the operator has addressed the hard and soft tissue structures that make up the framework and house the neurovascular structures of the body, it is now appropriate to investigate the visceral field by following the base-up, centre-out principle. The following discussion will provide an introduction to the long lever approach when treating the viscera.

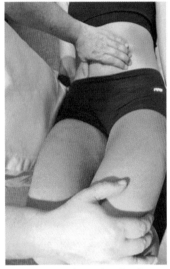

FIG 5.1: *Hand position for the general visceral treatment.*

The operator brings the patient's knees and hips into flexion bilaterally so that the patient's feet are flat on the table. This brings their anterior abdominal wall off tension and makes the area easier to palpate, the legs a more effective lever for the operator, and the patient more comfortable. With his downtable hand at the knees to control the movement of the lever, the operator places his uptable hand on the abdomen so that his thumb beds and fingertips are interacting with the lateral aspects of the ascending and descending colon (**FIG 5.1**).

The uptable hands will act as short counter-levers on the viscera so that the movement of the legs is a rhythmic oscillation of the long lever. Together, the short and long levers will create a push/pull force that either meets, opposes, or encourages motion at the viscera, whether through a balanced, direct, or indirect approach. In other words, as the legs move in one direction, the operator can move the abdomen in the same direction, create a fixed point at the abdomen, or, to generate even more tension, move it in the opposite direction of the lever. For example, if the operator wanted to treat

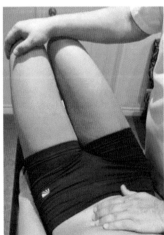

FIG 5.2

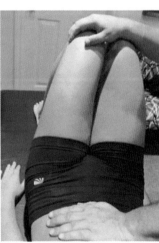

FIG 5.3

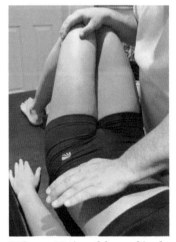

FIG 5.4: *Motion of the combined levers.* The motion at the long and short levers are in opposition to one another, as supplemented from FIG 5.3.

Using counter-leverage through a combined short and long lever. In this example, the operator is generating tension using both the legs as long levers as well as his hand as a short lever and fulcrum.

directly, he would move the levers to the patient's left while inducing traction laterally at the abdomen to the right (**FIG 5.2 - 5.5**). The way that the operator utilizes the leverage to approach the barrier will depend, as always, on the patient and the lesion pattern they present.

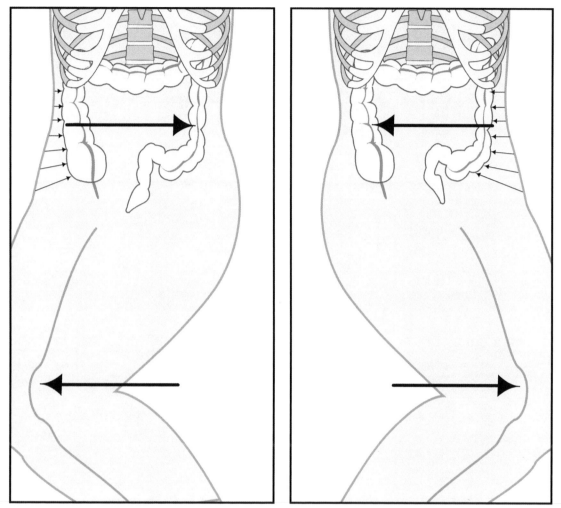

FIG 5.5: *Using leverage to treat the abdominal viscera.* To treat directly, the operator creates a fixed point and draws the colon off of the wall of the abdomen while moving the levers in the opposite direction.

Autonomic Innervation Abdominal and Pelvic Viscera: Sympathetic ANS

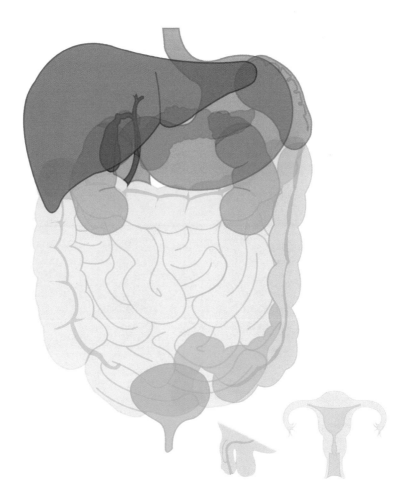

FIG 5.6: *Innervation of the abdominal viscera through the sympathetic autonomic nervous system.*

Considerations:
The postsynaptic nerve fibers travel via peri-arterial plexuses around branches of the abdominal aorta.

The presynaptic axons of the greater, lesser and least splanchnic nerves pass through the respiratory diaphragm and thus may be affected by mechanical lesions at the D/L junction. Lumber splanchnic nerves may also be affected since the spinal segment origin is located approximately four segments above the corresponding vertebral segment.

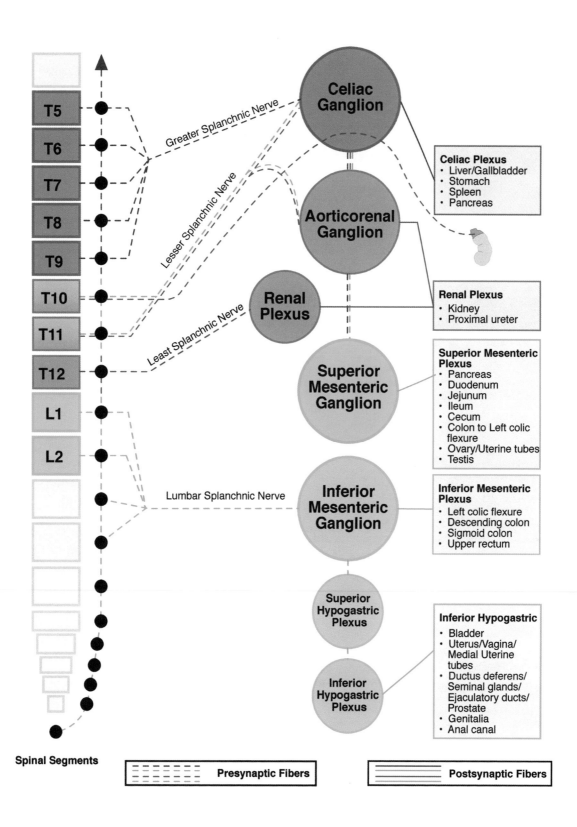

Spinal Segments

Presynaptic Fibers

Postsynaptic Fibers

Autonomic Innervation Abdominal and Pelvic Viscera: Parasympathetic ANS

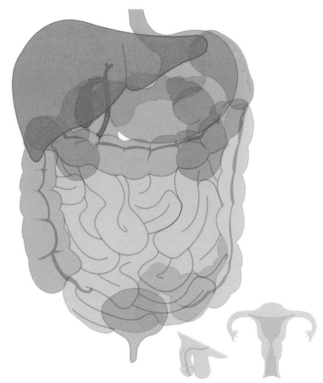

Pathway of Vagus Nerve (CNX)

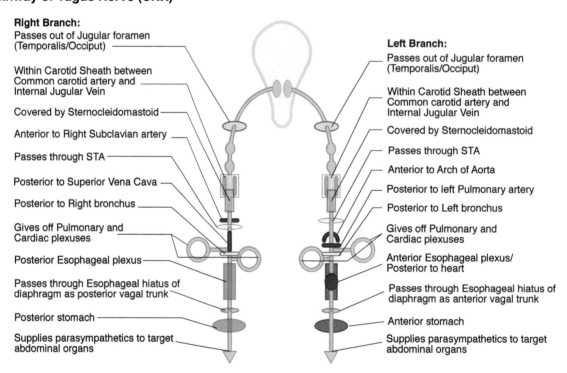

Right Branch:

Passes out of Jugular foramen (Temporalis/Occiput)

Within Carotid Sheath between Common carotid artery and Internal Jugular Vein

Covered by Sternocleidomastoid

Anterior to Right Subclavian artery

Passes through STA

Posterior to Superior Vena Cava

Posterior to Right bronchus

Gives off Pulmonary and Cardiac plexuses

Posterior Esophageal plexus

Passes through Esophageal hiatus of diaphragm as posterior vagal trunk

Posterior stomach

Supplies parasympathetics to target abdominal organs

Left Branch:

Passes out of Jugular foramen (Temporalis/Occiput)

Within Carotid Sheath between Common carotid artery and Internal Jugular Vein

Covered by Sternocleidomastoid

Passes through STA

Anterior to Arch of Aorta

Posterior to left Pulmonary artery

Posterior to Left bronchus

Gives off Pulmonary and Cardiac plexuses

Anterior Esophageal plexus/ Posterior to heart

Passes through Esophageal hiatus of diaphragm as anterior vagal trunk

Anterior stomach

Supplies parasympathetics to target abdominal organs

FIG 5.7(a): *Innervation of the abdominal viscera through the parasympathetic autonomic nervous system.*

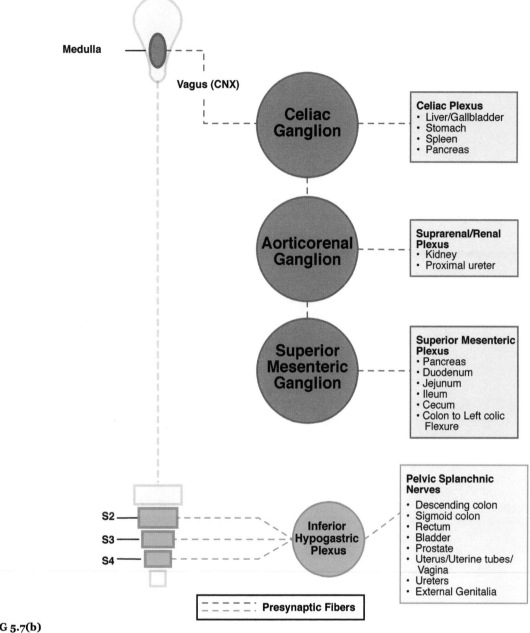

Medulla

Vagus (CNX)

Celiac Ganglion

Celiac Plexus
- Liver/Gallbladder
- Stomach
- Spleen
- Pancreas

Aorticorenal Ganglion

Suprarenal/Renal Plexus
- Kidney
- Proximal ureter

Superior Mesenteric Ganglion

Superior Mesenteric Plexus
- Pancreas
- Duodenum
- Jejunum
- Ileum
- Cecum
- Colon to Left colic Flexure

S2
S3
S4

Inferior Hypogastric Plexus

Pelvic Splanchnic Nerves
- Descending colon
- Sigmoid colon
- Rectum
- Bladder
- Prostate
- Uterus/Uterine tubes/ Vagina
- Ureters
- External Genitalia

= = = = = : **Presynaptic Fibers**

FIG 5.7(b)

Arterial Branches of the Abdominal Aorta (Sites of potential obstruction)

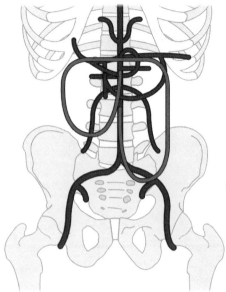

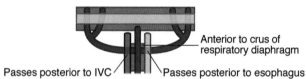

Anterior to crus of
respiratory diaphragm

Passes posterior to IVC

Passes posterior to esophagus

Inferior Phrenic Artery
- Approximate level of T12
- Retroperitoneal

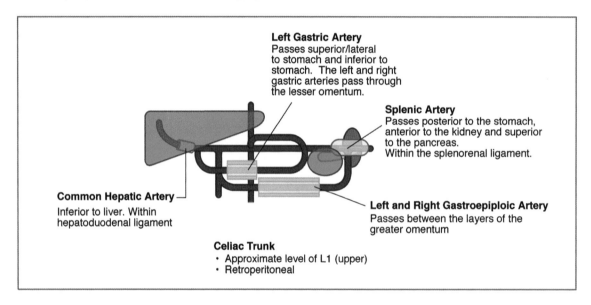

Left Gastric Artery
Passes superior/lateral
to stomach and inferior to
stomach. The left and right
gastric arteries pass through
the lesser omentum.

Splenic Artery
Passes posterior to the stomach,
anterior to the kidney and superior
to the pancreas.
Within the splenorenal ligament.

Common Hepatic Artery
Inferior to liver. Within
hepatoduodenal ligament

Left and Right Gastroepiploic Artery
Passes between the layers of the
greater omentum

Celiac Trunk
- Approximate level of L1 (upper)
- Retroperitoneal

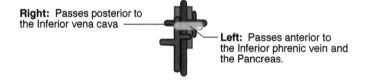

Right: Passes posterior to
the Inferior vena cava

Left: Passes anterior to
the Inferior phrenic vein and
the Pancreas.

Middle Suprarenal Artery
- Approximate level of L1
- Passes anterior to crus of diaphragm

FIG 5.8(a)

* Note: Not all branches of the abdominal aorta are represented here.

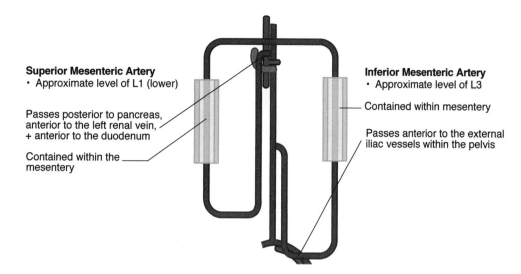

Superior Mesenteric Artery
• Approximate level of L1 (lower)

Passes posterior to pancreas, anterior to the left renal vein, + anterior to the duodenum

Contained within the mesentery

Inferior Mesenteric Artery
• Approximate level of L3

Contained within mesentery

Passes anterior to the external iliac vessels within the pelvis

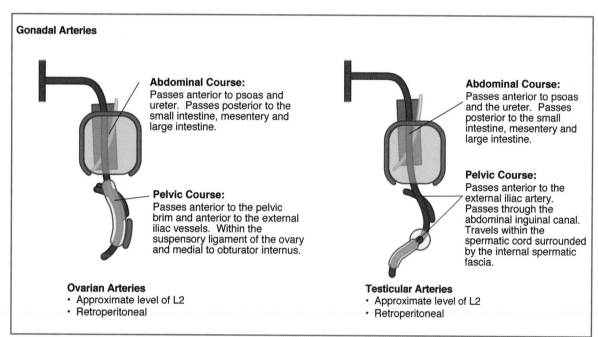

Gonadal Arteries

Abdominal Course:
Passes anterior to psoas and ureter. Passes posterior to the small intestine, mesentery and large intestine.

Pelvic Course:
Passes anterior to the pelvic brim and anterior to the external iliac vessels. Within the suspensory ligament of the ovary and medial to obturator internus.

Ovarian Arteries
• Approximate level of L2
• Retroperitoneal

Abdominal Course:
Passes anterior to psoas and the ureter. Passes posterior to the small intestine, mesentery and large intestine.

Pelvic Course:
Passes anterior to the external iliac artery. Passes through the abdominal inguinal canal. Travels within the spermatic cord surrounded by the internal spermatic fascia.

Testicular Arteries
• Approximate level of L2
• Retroperitoneal

Passes anterior to crus of diaphragm

Right: Passes posterior to the inferior vena cava, duodenum and right inferior suprarenal vein. Anterior to right ureter.

Left: Passes posterior to the pancreas, omental bursa, left inferior suprarenal vein. Anterior to the left ureter.

Renal Arteries
• Approximate level between L1 and L2
• Retroperitoneal

FIG 5.8(b)

* Note: Not all branches of the abdominal aorta are represented here.

Venous Tributaries to the Systemic Venous Return (Sites of potential obstruction)

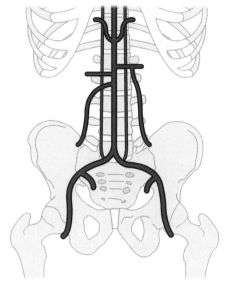

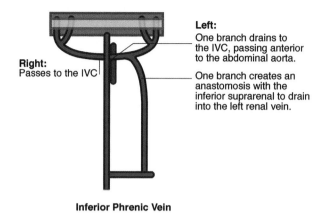

Left:
One branch drains to the IVC, passing anterior to the abdominal aorta.

One branch creates an anastomosis with the inferior suprarenal to drain into the left renal vein.

Right:
Passes to the IVC

Inferior Phrenic Vein

Passes anterior to crus of diaphragm

Right: Passes posterior to the duodenum. anterior to the right ureter.

Left: Anterior to the left ureter. Receives tributaries from the left inferior phrenic vein and left gonadal vein.

Renal Veins

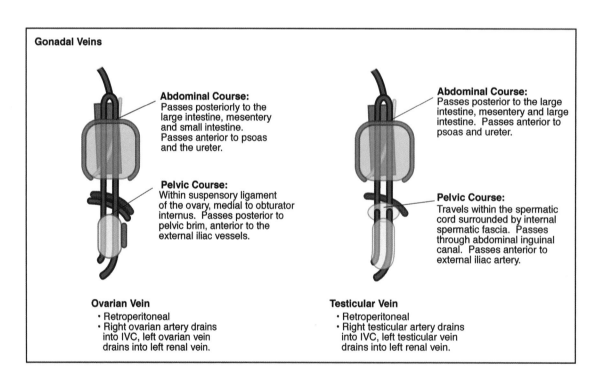

Gonadal Veins

Abdominal Course:
Passes posteriorly to the large intestine, mesentery and small intestine. Passes anterior to psoas and the ureter.

Pelvic Course:
Within suspensory ligament of the ovary, medial to obturator internus. Passes posterior to pelvic brim, anterior to the external iliac vessels.

Ovarian Vein
• Retroperitoneal
• Right ovarian artery drains into IVC, left ovarian vein drains into left renal vein.

Abdominal Course:
Passes posterior to the large intestine, mesentery and large intestine. Passes anterior to psoas and ureter.

Pelvic Course:
Travels within the spermatic cord surrounded by internal spermatic fascia. Passes through abdominal inguinal canal. Passes anterior to external iliac artery.

Testicular Vein
• Retroperitoneal
• Right testicular artery drains into IVC, left testicular vein drains into left renal vein.

FIG 5.9   * Note: Not all venous tributaries of systemic circulation within the abdomen are represented here.

Venous Tributaries to the Portal Venous Return (Sites of potential obstruction)

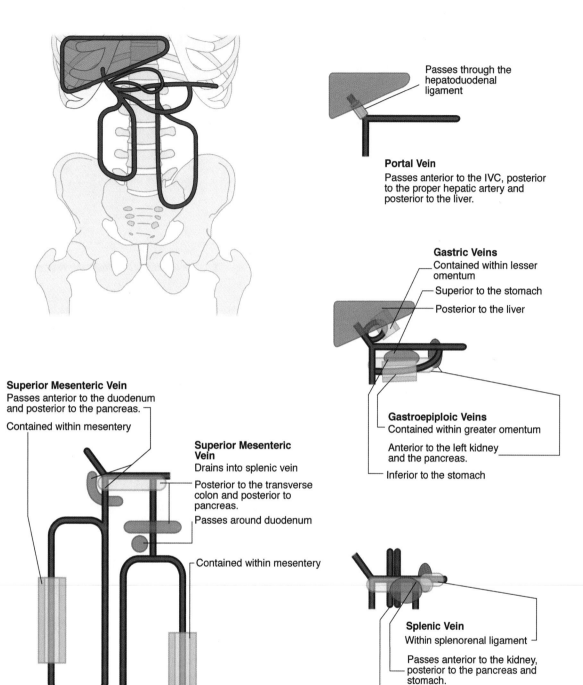

Passes through the hepatoduodenal ligament

Portal Vein
Passes anterior to the IVC, posterior to the proper hepatic artery and posterior to the liver.

Gastric Veins
Contained within lesser omentum
Superior to the stomach
Posterior to the liver

Gastroepiploic Veins
Contained within greater omentum
Anterior to the left kidney and the pancreas.
Inferior to the stomach

Superior Mesenteric Vein
Passes anterior to the duodenum and posterior to the pancreas.
Contained within mesentery

Superior Mesenteric Vein
Drains into splenic vein
Posterior to the transverse colon and posterior to pancreas.
Passes around duodenum
Contained within mesentery

Splenic Vein
Within splenorenal ligament
Passes anterior to the kidney, posterior to the pancreas and stomach.
Passes anterior to the abdominal aorta and the IVC

FIG 5.10   * Note: Not all venous tributaries of the portal system are represented here.

Lymphatic Drainage of the Abdominal Viscera

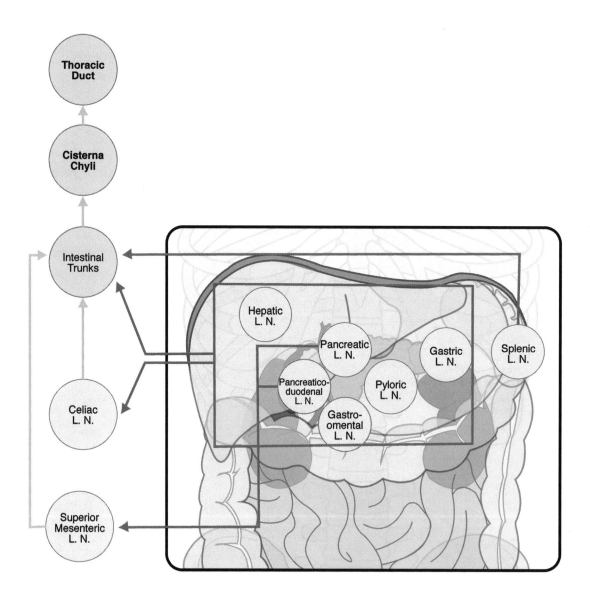

FIG 5.11(a)

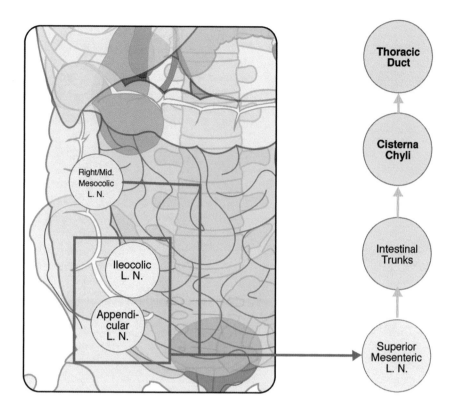

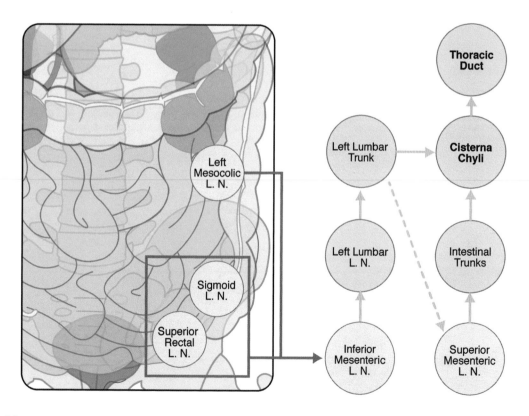

FIG 5.11(b)

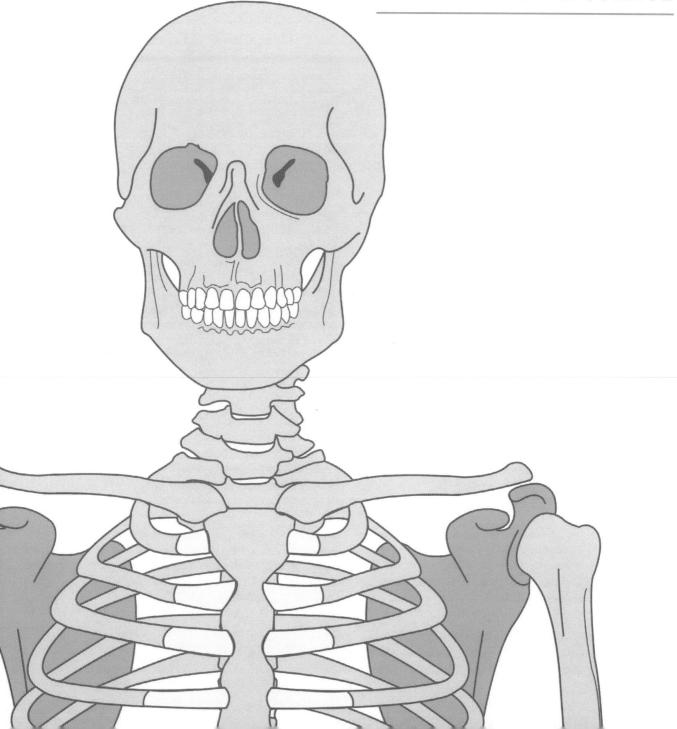

CHAPTER SIX

SYNTHESIZING THE SCIENCE

Synthesizing the Science

Time will be taken at this point to examine some of the scientific concepts that underpin the probable mechanisms of action with respect to osteopathic treatment. The concepts to be covered are mechanotransduction, vasomotion, and axoplasmic flow.

Mechanotransduction

Prior to examining mechanotransduction, a synthesized definition will be provided for contextual purposes. The term refers to:

> *The process of converting mechanical loads into biochemical signals that modulate a variety of cellular functions.*

The scientific understanding of mechanotransduction is constantly evolving. The general consensus among researchers in the field is that mechanical signals will interact with mechanisms that control cell shape and structure, as well as many intracellular functions.

Some research points to consistent disturbance to vascular flow in a manner that leads to vascular dysfunction. This disturbance is related, in part, to mechanical activation of endothelial cells. Clinically, for the operator, this provides a probable mechanism of action with respect to the osteopathic lesion and vascular dysfunction. If there is a lack of expected tissue mobility (bone tissue, articular elements, ligaments, tendons, muscles, etc.), then there is likely mechanical disturbance to the vascular elements in relation to the tissue. If the lack of tissue mobility (i.e., osteopathic lesion) is present for a long period of time, then the current research suggests that mechanical disturbance will cause vascular disease. Considering the mechanistic relationship between disturbed blood flow and vascular disease through the endothelial cells, there is a strong case to be made for improving tissue mobility to reduce mechanical challenges to vascular elements.

Further research verifies that pressure-dependent myogenic resistance arteries present mechanically gated ion channels as the main regulator of smooth muscle tone. It is also noted that dysfunction in the mechanically gated ion channels is implicated in cardiac arrhythmia, cardiac hypertrophy, Duchenne muscular dystrophy, as well as various other cardiovascular diseases. The mechanically gated ion channels are examples of mechanotransduction in action as a control for physiological regulation. It has been highlighted here with respect to vascular physiology, however, that the same mechanisms are at play in other physiological processes.

The sense of hearing is based on changing mechanical information into a cellular signal. Many sensory nerves take mechanical information and turn it into an action potential that will then lead to a cellular response on the other end of the nerve. The mechanically gated membrane channels existing in pressure-dependent myogenic resistance arteries are present in other cells. Essentially, they open or close to transport materials between the internal and external environments of the cell (primarily ions). There is a strong scientific understanding that mechanical information controls many functions within the human organism. Because of this strong understanding, there is a case to be made for normalization of abnormal mechanical forces as essential to the normal homeostatic functions of a human organism. It is the imperative of the osteopathic operator to examine a patient and synthesize the understanding of mechanics, functional anatomy, and functional physiology. It is the operator's obligation, moreover, to locate any mechanical issues and remove them; the goal is to facilitate normal function and health of the human organism.

Vasomotion

The general theme of many osteopathic conversations about vasomotion is that it is mediated in the medulla oblongata; thus, there will often be treatment applied with respect to the occipito-atlantal joint in order to have some interface with what is termed the 'chief vasomotor center' (VMC). The concept of the VMC was first conceived by Filipp Ovsyannikov in 1871. Further scientific investigation does not support the concept of a single VMC. Instead, the current understanding is that, in various parts of the brain and brain stem, there is a presympathetic network of neurons that regulate vascular tone throughout the body. To be clear, this means that there is not one single location for control of vasomotion. This also means that we are speaking about vascular tone, not specified regulation of individual blood vessels at the level of the brain or brain stem.

The aforementioned conversation seems to have stalled in some areas of the world. No further progress has been made past the mechanism for vasomotion proposed by Filipp Ovsyannikov in 1871, and accepted by the contemporaneous scientific community. It is of use to look to the progress that scientific investigation has made since 1871 with respect to vasomotion and regulation of blood flow locally and systemically. Attention to new research needs to be paid particularly to fill the void in osteopathic knowledge. To fill this void, it will be explained below that the current scientific understanding of vasomotion is independent of the nervous system, heart rate, and respiratory rate.

To provide an examination of the current scientific understanding of vasomotion, it will be made clear that, at present, there is no single accepted mechanism for the regulation of blood flow in a given area. There are three widely accepted mechanisms that do have general scientific confidence and are being further investigated. Those three possible mechanisms are as follows:

1. Oscillatory release of intracellular calcium (within the cellular components of the actual blood vessel)

2. Oscillatory release of calcium in the sarcolemma (the muscular portion of the blood vessel)

3. Oscillations in glycolysis (within the cellular components of the actual blood vessel)

As these three mechanisms are still under investigation, the best statement that can be made from an osteopathic standpoint is this: regardless of the specific mechanism, blood flow has auto-regulatory capabilities. It is crucial to recognize that blood, moreover, will regulate based on the inputs available to it. Considering the discussion in the mechanotransduction section of this chapter, which points to mechanically gated ion channels in pressure-dependent myogenic resistance arteries, it is possible to consider those channels in relation to mechanical disturbances to the endothelial lining of blood vessels (even though that relationship has not yet been fully explored). Clinically speaking, the osteopathic operator has an opportunity to remove mechanical inputs that will impact the endothelial lining of the blood vessels (as described when discussing mechanotransduction), and that will also likely affect the auto-regulatory mechanisms controlling vasomotion.

Axoplasmic Flow

Axoplasmic flow is the commonly used term in many osteopathic circles. Currently, the term 'axonal transport' is used interchangeably with 'axonal flow' in scientific discussion. Regardless of the term applied, the concept relates to the movement of substances along a nerve. Axoplasm is the cytoplasm inside of an axon; various cellular materials will move through it to aid functioning of the entire nerve cell. The movement of these materials is classified as anterograde (from the nerve cell body out to the axon) and retrograde (from the axon to the nerve cell body). Both anterograde and retrograde flow are accomplished by carrier mechanisms (kinesins and dyneins). The carrier mechanisms move along microtubules that run the length of the axon and are formed by tubulin. Anterograde flow is further broken down into *fast axonal transport* and *slow axonal transport*. The characteristics of both are as follows:

1. Fast Axonal Transport – there is consistent movement of the carrying mechanism. This mechanism is transporting proteins that are comparatively smaller than those moved by *slow axonal transport* and these proteins are generally destined for structures in the membrane of the axon (such as ion channels).

2. Slow Axonal Transport – the movement of the carrying mechanism is not actually slow. It presents pauses in order to offload the comparatively larger proteins being transported, which are generally destined for structures in the cytoplasm and the cytoskeleton (such as organelles).

Retrograde flow is characterized as follows:

1. The substances transported from the axon to the nerve cell body to be presented to lysosomes and other clean-up processes. The actual substances transported are exogenous substances, old membrane constituents, and trophic factors.

2. Due to the generally larger size of the materials being transported in retrograde flow, it tends to be slower based on physical drag caused by the size of the materials.

When considering that movement of essential proteins and other substances between the nerve cell body and the axon is necessary for proper maintenance of nerve function, it is important to research the processes that may interfere with this function. There is information produced through animal models that shows changes in axonal transport when pressure is applied to the nerve under scrutiny. The overarching observation among the studies is that there *are* changes in function of axonal transport with pressure changes, and then related changes in function of the structure being supplied by that nerve. As most of the studies are performed in animal models, one must speculate in order to apply the scientific data to human anatomy; however, it is worth noting that the mechanisms at play in the animal models are analogs for the mechanisms in humans. Considering that there are parallels to be drawn between the animal models and human physiology, we can hypothesize that abnormal and sustained pressure on a nerve will alter axonal transport, nerve health, and function of the structure being supplied by the nerve.

Connecting the Science

There is enough information present in the scientific literature to show that abnormal mechanical pressure will alter function of various structures in the body. It is known that there are clear changes to endothelial function in blood vessels with long-term mechanical disturbance of blood flow. Moreover, local auto-regulation of blood flow relies on *mechanically gated ion channels*, which means that local increases in external pressure can interfere with vascular function. In addition, because axonal transport is affected by pressure in animal models, it is reasonable to hypothesize that the same is true in humans. Therefore, we can posit that the lack of dynamic mobility in a structure that is the hallmark of the osteopathic lesion affects the physiological processes in the direct (and indirect) area of the lesion. The long-term lack of dynamic mobility affecting the control mechanisms for physiological processes (noted above) influence long-term health of the specific lesion area, as well as other interconnected areas, over time. The processes noted are all auto-regulatory, according to the inputs they depend on to make decisions to alter function as needed. When the input needed to control the auto-regulatory process is mechanical and there is a long-term mechanical change (e.g., an osteopathic lesion develops), there will be some effect on the function and health of the process.

Looking back to early osteopathic literature, we can argue that the clinical observations presented by the early operators point to the mechanical interruption of functions as significant challenges to patient health. It is also possible to see improvements of patient health when the mechanical interruptions to functions are removed. This removal technique is related to the auto-regulation of many functions based on mechanical inputs. In the case of the discoverer of Osteopathy, Dr. Andrew Taylor Still, relationships between mechanical discord and health become palpable when reviewing passages from *Philosophy and Mechanical Principles of Osteopathy*.

The following is an important excerpt that explains the necessity of beginning with the mechanical (empirical observation) to treat the whole:

An Osteopath, in his search for the cause of diseases, starts out to find the mechanical cause. He feels that the people expect more than guessing of an osteopath. He feels that he must put his hand on the cause and prove what he says by what he does; that he will not get off by the feeble-minded trash of stale habits that go with doctors of medicine. By his knowledge he must show his ability to go beyond the musty bread of symptomatology.

Further evidence of Dr. Still's observation of the link between mechanical discord, physiological control mechanisms, and health can be found in *Philosophy of Osteopathy* when he writes:

> The Osteopath seeks first physiological perfection of form, by normally adjusting the osseous frame work, so that all arteries may deliver blood to nourish and construct all parts. Also that the veins may carry away all impurities dependent upon them for renovation. Also that the nerves of all classes may be free and unobstructed while applying the powers of life and motion to all divisions, and the whole system of nature's laboratory.

To be clear, Dr. Still had not been exposed to the specific science of how Mechanotransduction, Vasomotion, and Axoplasmic Flow/Axonal Transport are modified by mechanical forces. However, he had clinically observed that those mechanisms *did* exist and that he was able to interface with them while not having seen the specific science that is currently available. It can be further argued that, when examining his writings, Dr. Still was clearly able to observe the auto-regulatory mechanisms in action. The observation of auto-regulatory mechanisms in relation to mechanical discord is palpable when Dr. Still writes the following in *Philosophy of Osteopathy*:

> You as Osteopathic machinists can go no farther than to adjust the abnormal condition, in which you find the afflicted. Nature will do the rest.

Further evidence of the observation between mechanical discord and alterations in physiological function is visible when Dr. Still says the following in *Philosophy of Osteopathy*:

> The Osteopath reasons if he reasons at all, that order and health are inseparable, and that when order in all parts is found, disease cannot prevail, and if order is complete and disease should be found, there is no use for order. And if order and health are universally one in union, then the doctor cannot usefully, physiologically, or philosophically be guided by any scale of reason, otherwise.

Looking to *Philosophy and Mechanical Principles of Osteopathy* we see even more evidence of the observational understanding of auto-regulatory mechanisms:

> If you allow yourself to reason at all, you must know that sensation must be normal and always on guard to give notice by local or general misery of unnatural accumulation of the circulating fluids. Every nerve must be free to act and do its part. Your duty as a master mechanic is to know that the engine is kept in a perfect condition, so that there will be no functional disturbance to any nerve, or vein, or artery that supplies and governs

the skin, the fascia, the muscle, the blood, or any fluid that should be in free circulation to sustain life and renovate the system from deposits that would cause what we call disease.

In the quotation above, Dr. Still is referencing the relationship between altered dynamic mechanical function (a.k.a., "functional disturbance") to nerves, arteries, or veins and disease states. At the time of writing this work there was a deepening understanding of the actual mechanical components at play in relation to what Andrew Taylor Still noted in the period of mid-1860s until his death in 1917. It is the clinical evidence and observation of Dr. Still that guides the osteopathic operator to understand that mechanical discord will influence auto-regulatory processes, and current science further proves this natural principle.

When placing Osteopathic Manual Practice in today's scientific framework, it is often stated that doing a randomized control trial is difficult with respect to treatment and outcomes. This is true when attempting to map treatment application directly onto responsive outcomes. It is much more useful to look at the actual physiological control mechanisms presented within the human body, as well as that which will interfere with them. There is mounting evidence that many physiological processes are dependent on mechanical input and, as such, will be altered by changes in mechanical input. Because this is the case, we must ensure that all mechanical inputs are functioning in the appropriate manner, as they are essential to the normal auto-regulation of all body mechanics.

AFTERWORD & APPENDIX

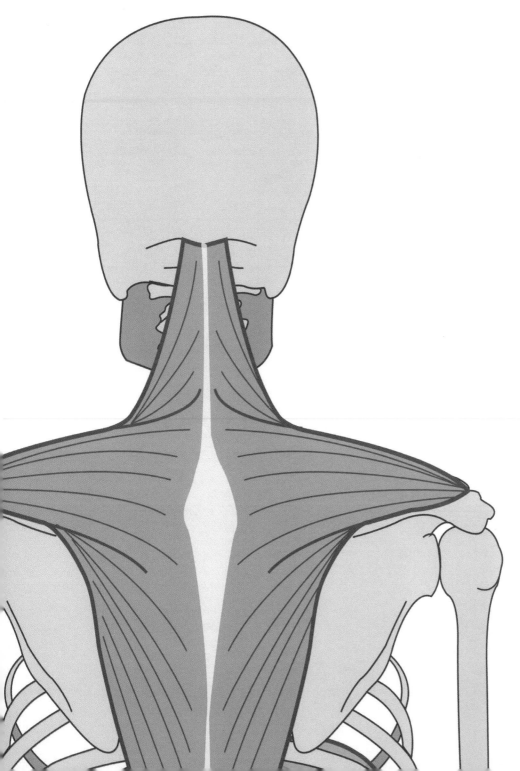

Afterword

In closing, the author hopes that this book has been an effective means of discussing an approach to general osteopathic treatment. This book was written to provide an introductory understanding of treatment applications, body mechanics from an osteopathic perspective, and the role of general treatment within osteopathic practice. This book is not intended to be the lone authority on general treatment, nor is it a how-to manual of technique. The author understands that this is but one approach, based on the concepts and principles of Osteopathy set forth by Dr. Andrew Taylor Still, to delivering general treatment. In essence, what has been offered can be augmented from practitioner to practitioner. Every attempt has been made to illustrate these unwavering principles to prospective readers so that they may have a foundation upon which to base their own general treatment. If these concepts and principles are clearly understood, then the practitioner should be capable of applying general treatment from any position, on any patient, in any circumstance, while acknowledging that treatment will manifest differently each time. If the reader is cognizant of these ideas, then the book has been successful in its intentions.

Appendix

The following table is a summary of anatomical information obtained from *Gray's Anatomy 32nd Edition* and *Thieme Atlas of Anatomy*. It is provided only as a reference to additional information relevant to this handbook, and as a supplement to further study.

Muscle	Attachment Points	Action	Innervation
Pelvic Floor			
Iliococcygeus (part of the levator ani)	Tendinous arch of the levator ani to the coccyx	Supports pelvic viscera and help move coccyx; puborectalis maintains anorectal fascia and canal	Pudendal (S2-S4) (and coccygeal plexus for coccygeus)
Pubococcygeus (part of the levator ani)	Pubis, lateral to puborectalis, to the coccyx		
Puborectalis (part of the levator ani)	Pubis to opposite pubis on either side of the pubic symphysis wrapping around rectum		
Coccygeus	Ischial spine to the coccyx and sacrum		
Deep transverse perineal (*Note: the external urethral sphincter is a division of the deep transverse perineal)	Inferior pubic ramus and ischial ramus to the wall of vagina or prostate and central tendon; external urethral sphincter encircles the urethra	Supports pelvic organs; closes the urethra	
Superficial transverse perineal	Ischial ramus to central tendon		
External anal sphincter	Central tendon to anococcygeal ligament	Closes the anus	
Bulbospongiosus	Central tendon to the clitoris or penile raphe	Narrows vaginal introitus or surrounds corpus spongiosum	
Ischiocavernosus	Ischial ramus to crus of penis or clitoris	Squeezes blood into corpus cavernous of penis or clitoris	
Lateral rotators of the hip			
Piriformis	Anterior surface of the sacrum to the greater trochanter	Laterally rotates hip	Nerve to piriformis (S1-S2)
Superior gemellus	Ischial spine to the intertrochanteric fossa		Nerve to obturator internus (L5-S2)
Obturator internus	Internal surface of obturator foramen and membrane to the greater trochanter		
Inferior gemellus	Ischial tuberosity to the intertrochanteric fossa		Nerve to quadratus femoris (L4-S1)
Quadratus femoris	Ischial tuberosity to the quadrate tubercle and intertrochanteric crest		
Obturator externus	External surface of obturator foramen and membrane to the trochanteric fossa		Obturator (L2-L4)

Muscle	Attachment Points	Action	Innervation
Quadriceps Femoris			
Rectus femoris	AIIS and notch below to the base of the tibial tuberosity via patellar tendon	Flexes hip; extends knee	Femoral (L2-L4)
Vastus lateralis	Greater trochanter and lateral lip of linea aspera to the tibial tuberosity via patellar tendon	Extends knee	Femoral (L2-L4)
Vastus intermedius	Anterior shaft of the femur to the tibial tuberosity via patellar tendon		
Vastus medialis	Intertrochanteric line and medial lip of linea aspera to the tibial tuberosity via patellar tendon		
Hip Flexors			
Sartorius	ASIS and inferior notch to the tibial pes anserine insertion (anteriorly)	Flexes, abducts, and laterally rotates thigh at hip; flexes knee	
Psoas (major and minor)	Transverse processes, bodies, and intervertebral discs of lumbar vertebrae to the lesser trochanter	Flexes, abducts, and laterally rotates thigh at hip	Femoral (L2-4) and lumbar spinal nerves
Iliacus	Iliac crest and fossa to the lesser trochanter		
Hip Adductors			
Adductor longus	Body of pubis, inferior to pubic crest, to middle third of linea aspera	Adducts hip	Obturator (L2-L4)
Adductor brevis	Body and inferior ramus of pubis to the pectineal line and proximal third of linea aspera		
Adductor magnus	Inferior ramus of pubis, ischial ramus, and ischial tuberosity to gluteal tuberosity, linea aspera, supracondylar line, and adductor tubercle	Adducts hip (adductor portion); extends hip (hamstring portion)	Obturator (L2-L4) and sciatic (L4-S3)
Pectineus	Pectineal line of the pubis to the pectineal line of the femur	Adducts, flexes, and laterally rotates hip	Femoral and obturator (L2-L4)
Gracilis	Body and inferior ramus of pubis to tibial pes anserine insertion (medially)	Adducts, flexes, and medially rotates hip	Obturator (L2-L4)

Muscle	Attachment Points	Action	Innervation
Hip Extensors			
Biceps femoris	Ischial tuberosity (long head) and distal linea aspera (short head) to the fibular head	Extends hip; flexes and laterally rotates knee	Sciatic (L4-S3) and common peroneal (L4-S2)
Semimembranosus	Ischial tuberosity to the medial condyle of the tibia	Extends hip; flexes and medially rotates knee	Sciatic (L4-S3)
Semitendinosus	Ischial tuberosity to the tibial pes anserine insertion (posteriorly)		
Gluteus maximus	Iliac crest, dorsal surface of the sacrum and coccyx, and sacrotuberous ligament to the IT band (lateral condyle of the tibia) and gluteal tuberosity	Extends and laterally rotates hip	Inferior gluteal (L5-S2)
Hip Abductors			
Tensor Fascia Latae	ASIS and iliac crest to the IT band (lateral condyle of the tibia)	Tensor fascia lata; abducts and flexes hip and knee	Superior gluteal (L4-S1)
Gluteus medius	External surface of the ilium, superiorly, to the greater trochanter	Abducts and medially rotates hip	
Gluteus minimus	External surface of the ilium, inferiorly, to the greater trochanter		
Anterior Compartment of Lower Leg			
Tibialis anterior	Lateral condyle of the tibia to the medial cuneiform and 1st metatarsal	Dorsiflexion and inversion of the ankle	Deep peroneal (L4-S2)
Extensor digitorum longus	Lateral condyle of tibia, interosseous membrane, and anterior surface of fibula to the phalanges of the lateral 4 digits	Dorsiflexion and eversion of the ankle; extends lateral 4 digits	
Extensor hallucis longus	Anterior surface of fibula and interosseous membrane to the distal phalanx of the hallux	Dorsiflexion of the ankle; extends hallux	
Peroneus tertius	Distal third of fibula and interosseous membrane to the 5th metatarsal	Dorsiflexion of the ankle; eversion	

Muscle	Attachment Points	Action	Innervation
Lateral compartment of the lower limb			
Peroneus longus	Head and proximal lateral surface of fibula to the 1st metatarsal and medial cuneiform	Plantarflexion and eversion of the ankle	Superficial peroneal (L4-S2)
Peroneus brevis	Distal two thirds of the lateral surface of the fibula to the 5th metatarsal		
Posterior compartment of the lower limb (superficial)			
Gastrocnemius	Lateral and medial condyles of the femur to the calcaneal tuberosity via calcaneal tendon	Plantarflexion of the ankle; flexes knee	Tibial (L4-S3)
Plantaris	Lateral supracondylar line of the femur to the calcaneal tuberosity via calcaneal tendon		
Soleus	Head and posterior surface of the fibula and soleal line to the calcaneal tuberosity via calcaneal tendon	Plantarflexion of the ankle	
Posterior compartment of the lower limb (deep)			
Popliteus	Lateral epicondyle of femur to the posterior surface of the tibia	Flexes and 'unlocks' knee from extension	
Tibialis posterior	Posterior surface of tibia, interosseous membrane, and fibula to the navicular, cuneiform, cuboid, and bases of 2nd through 4th metatarsals	Plantarflexion and inversion of the ankle	
Flexor digitorum longus	Posterior surface of the tibia to the distal phalanges of the lateral 4 digits	Flexes lateral 4 digits; plantarflexion of the ankle	Tibial (L4-S3)
Flexor hallucis longus	Distal two thirds of the posterior surface of the fibula and interosseous membrane to the distal phalanx of the hallux	Flexes hallux; plantarflexion of the ankle	
Intrinsic muscles of the foot			
Extensor digitorum brevis	Calcaneus to the dorsal aponeurosis and middle phalanges of digits 2 through 4	Extends digits	Deep peroneal (L4-S2)
Extensor hallucis brevis	Calcaneus to dorsal aponeurosis and proximal phalanx of hallux	Extends hallux	

Muscle	Attachment Points	Action	Innervation
Abductor hallucis	Calcaneal tuberosity and plantar aponeurosis to proximal phalanx of hallus	Flexes hallux	Medial plantar (tibial)
Flexor hallucis brevis	Medial and intermediate cuneiform and plantar calcaneocuboid ligament to proximal phalanx via medial and lateral sesamoid	Flexes hallux	Medial and lateral plantar (tibial)
Adductor hallucis	Metatarsals of digits 2 through 4, cuboid, lateral cuneiform (oblique head) and metatarsophalangeal joints of digits 3 through 5 (transverse head) to the proximal phalanx of the hallux	Flexes and adducts hallux	Lateral plantar (tibial)
Abductor digiti minimi	Calcaneal tuberosity and plantar aponeurosis to proximal phalanx of the 5th digit and 5th metatarsal	Flexes and abducts 5th digit	
Flexor digiti minimi brevis	Metatarsal of 5th digit and long plantar ligament to the proximal phalanx of 5th digit	Flexes 5th digit	
Opponens digiti minimi	Long plantar ligament and tendon sheath of peroneus longus to 5th metatarsal	Opposes 5th digit	
Flexor digitorum brevis	Calcaneal tuberosity and plantar aponeurosis to middle phalanges of digits 2 through 5	Flexes digits 2 through 5	Medial plantar (tibial)
Quadratus plantae	Calcaneal tuberosity to lateral border of flexor digitorum longus tendon	Augments tension of flexor digitorum longus	Lateral plantar (tibial)
First through fourth lumbricals	Medial border of flexor digitorum longus to dorsal aponeurosis of digits 2 through 5	Flexes, extends, and adducts digits 2 through 5	Medial and lateral plantar (tibial)
First through third plantar interossei	Medial border of metatarsals 3 through 5 to proximal phalanges of those same digits	Flexes, extends, and abducts digits 2 through 4	Lateral plantar (tibial)
First through fourth dorsal interossei	By two heads from opposing sides of all metatarsals to the proximal phalange of those same digits	Flexes, extends, and abducts digits 2 through 4	

Muscle	Attachment Points	Action	Innervation
Intrinsic muscles of the spine			
Multifidus	Lamina of all vertebrae to the TPs or articular processes of all vertebrae inferior, from C2 to the sacrum but most prominent in the lumbar region	Bilaterally: extends spine Unilaterally: rotates spine contralaterally (multifidus also sidebends the spine ipsilaterally)	Spinal nerves from the surrounding segments
Rotatores (longus, brevis)	Lamina and SPs of the thoracic vertebrae to the TPs of 1 or 2 segments inferiorly		
Interspinales	Between SPs of adjacent vertebrae in all spinal regions, more prominent in the lumbar and cervical regions	Extends the spine	Spinal nerves from the surrounding segments
Intertransversarii	Between TPs of adjacent vertebrae in all spinal regions, more prominent in the lumbar (medial and lateral) and cervical (anterior and posterior)	Bilaterally: stabilize and extends cervical and lumbar spine Unilaterally: Sidebends the spine ipsilaterally	
Erector Spinae			
Iliocostalis (lumborum, thoracis, and cervicis)	Sacrum, thoracolumbar fascia, and iliac crest to the angles of all ribs and TPs of C4-C7	Bilateral: extends spine (and head) Unilateral: sidebends spine ipsilaterally (and head)	Dorsal rami of the spinal nerves from the surrounding segments
Longissimus (thoracis, cervicis, and capitis)	Sacrum, thoracolumbar fascia, SPs of lumbar vertebrae, TPs of thoracic vertebrae, articular pillars of C4-C7 vertebrae to the TPs of the lumbar vertebrae, 2-12 ribs between the tubercles and angles, the transverse processes of the cervical vertebrae, mastoid process of the occiput		
Spinalis (thoracis and cervicis)	SPs of T10-L3, T1-T2, and C5-C7 to the SPs of T2-T8 and C2-C5, spanning all vertebrae on the lateral aspect	Bilateral: extends spine (and head) Unilateral: sidebends spine ipsilaterally (and head)	Dorsal rami of the spinal nerves from the surrounding segments
Posterior Abdominal Wall			
Quadratus lumborum	Transverse process of lumbar vertebrae and 12th rib to the iliac crest	Bilaterally: extends spine; pulls 12th rib inferiorly Unilaterally: sidebends spine	T12-L2 spinal nerves

Muscle	Attachment Points	Action	Innervation
Anterior Abdominal Wall			
External obliques	External surfaces ribs 5-12 to linea alba, rectus sheath, pubic tubercle, and iliac crest	Compress and support abdomen and viscera; flex trunk	Lower intercostal, iliohypogastric, and inguinal nerves
Rectus abdominis	Costal cartilages 5-7 and xiphoid process to the pubic tubercle		T5-T12 spinal nerves
Internal obliques	Thoracolumbar fascia, iliac crest, and inguinal ligament to ribs 10-12, linea alba, rectus sheath, and the pubic tubercle		T7-L1 spinal nerves, iliohypogastric and ilioinguinal nerves (T12-L1)
Transversus abdominis	Thoracolumbar fascia, iliac crest, ribs 7-12, ASIS, and the inguinal ligament to the linea alba and pubic tubercle	Compress and support abdomen and viscera; flex trunk	T7-L1 spinal nerves, iliohypogastric and ilioinguinal nerves (T12-L1)
Ventral and lateral surfaces of the trunk			
Pectoralis major	Sternal end of the clavicle and the sternocostal joints of ribs 1-7 to the greater tubercle of the humerus	Adducts, flexes, and medially rotates humerus	Medial (C8-T1) and lateral pectoral (C5-C7)
Pectoralis minor	Coracoid process to ribs 3-5	Stabilizes and anteriorizes scapula; raises ribs	
External intercostals	Superior border of one rib to the inferior border of inferior rib (obliquely, superolaterally to inferomedially) on the outer aspect of the rib cage	Elevates ribs during inhalation	Intercostal nerves T1-T11 (T2-T7 for transversus thoracis)
Transversus thoracis	Costal cartilages 2-6 to the xiphoid process on the inner surface of the rib cage	Depresses the ribs during exhalation	
Internal intercostals (*Note: innermost intercostals are regarded as a division of the internal intercostals)	Inferior border of one rib to the superior border of superior rib (obliquely, inferolaterally to superomedially) on the inner aspect of the rib cage	Depresses ribs during exhalation	Intercostal nerves T1-T11 (T2-T7 for transversus thoracis)
Serratus anterior	Ventral surface of the scapula to the lateral surface of ribs 1-8	Protracts and rotates scapula superiorly; elevates ribs	Long thoracic (C5-C7)
Diaphragm	Xiphoid process, inner surface of the lower six ribs, L1-L3 vertebral bodies and discs to the central tendon	Principal muscle of respiration and compressing abdominal viscera	Phrenic (C3-C5)

Muscle	Attachment Points	Action	Innervation
Dorsal surface of the trunk			
Trapezius	Nuchal line of the occiput, nuchal ligament, and SPs of the dorsal spine to the lateral third of the clavicle, acromion, and scapular spine in three portions (descending, transverse, and ascending)	Elevates, depresses, retracts, and rotates scapula	CNXI Spinal accessory (16) and cervical spinal nerves C2-C4
Latissimus dorsi	SPs of T6-T12, thoracolumbar fascia, iliac crest, and lower 4 ribs to the inferior angle of the scapula and intertubercular groove of the humerus	Extends, adducts, and medially rotates humerus	Thoracodorsal (C6-C8)
Serratus posterior inferior	Thoracolumbar fascia and SPs of T12-L3 to ribs 9-12 lateral to their angles	Depresses and draws ribs backwards	Intercostal nerves (T9-T12)
Serratus posterior superior	Nuchal ligament and SPs of C7-T3 to ribs 2-5 lateral to their angles	Elevates and draws ribs outwards	Intercostal nerves (T1-T5)
Levatores costarum (longus and brevis)	TPs of dorsal spine to the rib (one or two below) between its angle and tubercle	Bilaterally: extends thoracic spine Unilaterally: sidebends the thoracic spine ipsilateraly and rotates contralaterally; elevates ribs	Intercostal (spinal) nerves T1-T12
Shoulder girdle			
Rhomboid major and minor	Nuchal ligament and SPs of C7-T1 (minor) and T2-T5 (major) to the medial border of the scapula	Steadies, retracts, and rotates scapula	Dorsal scapular (C4-C5)
Levator scapulae	TPs of C1-C4 to the superior medial border of the scapula	Elevates scapula; sidebends neck ipsilaterally	Dorsal scapular (C4-C5)
Supraspinatus (part of the rotator cuff)	Supraspinous fossa to the greater tuberosity of the humerus	Abducts arm	Suprascapular (C4-C6)
Infraspinatus (part of the rotator cuff)	Infraspinous fossa to the greater tubercle of the humerus	Laterally rotates arm	
Subscapularis (part of the rotator cuff)	Subscapular fossa to the lesser tuberosity of the humerus	Medially rotates arm	Upper and lower subscapular (C5-C6)

Muscle	Attachment Points	Action	Innervation
Teres major	Inferior angle of the scapula to the inter-tubercular groove of the humerus	Adducts and medially rotates arm	Lower subscapular (C5-C6)
Teres minor (part of the rotator cuff)	Lateral border of the scapula to the greater tuberosity of the humerus	Laterally rotates and adducts arm	Axillary (C5-C6)
Deltoid	Lateral third of the clavicle, acromion, and scapular spine to the deltoid tuberosity of the humerus	Flexes and medially rotates arm; abducts arm, extends and laterally rotates arm	
Subclavius	First rib and its cartilage to the subclavian groove on the inferior aspect of the clavicle	Depresses and steadies clavicle	Subclavian nerve (C5-C6)
Anterior compartment of the arm			
Biceps brachii	Coracoid process (short head) and supraglenoid tubercle of the humerus (long head) to the radial tuberosity	Flexes arm and elbow; supinates forearm	Musculocutaneous (C5-C7)
Coracobrachialis	Coracoid process to the middle of the medial surface of the humerus	Flexes and adducts arm	
Brachialis	Distal, anterior half of the humerus to the coronoid process and ulnar tuberosity	Flexes forearm	
Posterior compartment of the arm			
Triceps brachii	Infraglenoid tubercle (long head) and on the humerus superior to (lateral head) and inferior to (medial head) radial groove to the olecranon	Extends and adducts arm; adducts forearm	Radial (C5-T1)
Anconeus	Lateral epicondyle of the humerus to the olecranon and posterior ulna	Extends forearm	

Muscle	Attachment Points	Action	Innervation
Superficial extensor compartment of the forearm			
Extensor carpi ulnaris	Lateral condyle of the humerus and posterior ulna to the base of the 5th metacarpal	Extends and adducts hand	Radial (C5-T1)
Extensor carpi radialis longus	Lateral supracondylar ridge of the humerus to the base of the 2nd metacarpal	Extends and abducts wrist	
Extensor carpi radialis brevis	Lateral epicondyle of the humerus to the base of the 3rd metacarpal		
Extensor digitorum	Lateral epicondyle of the humerus to the medial 4 digits	Extends wrist and medial 4 digits	
Brachioradialis	Lateral supracondylar ridge of the humerus to the styloid process of the radius	Flexes elbow and helps in pronation	
Deep extensor compartment of the forearm			
Extensor digiti minimi	Lateral epicondyle of the humerus to the 5th digit	Extends wrist and 5th digit	
Extensor indicis	Posterior ulna and interosseous membrane to the 2nd digit	Extends wrist and 2nd digit	
Extensor pollicis longus	Posterior ulna and interosseous membrane to the distal phalanx of the pollex	Extends and abducts wrist and pollex	Radial (C5-T1)
Extensor pollicis brevis	Posterior radius and interosseous membrane to the proximal phalanx of the pollex		
Intrinsic muscles of the hand			
Abductor pollicis brevis	Scaphoid, trapezium, and flexor retinaculum to the proximal phalanx of the pollex	Abducts pollex	Median (C5-T1)
Adductor pollicis	Palmar surface of 3rd metacarpal, capitate, and base of 2nd metacarpal to the proximal phalanx of pollex	Opposition and flexion of the pollex	Ulnar (C8-T1)
Flexor pollicis brevis	Flexor retinaculum, capitate, and trapezium to the proximal phalanx of the pollex		Median (C5-T1) and ulnar (C8-T1)
Opponens pollicis	Trapezium to the 1st metacarpal	Opposition of the pollex	Median (C5-T1)

Muscle	Attachment Points	Action	Innervation
Abductor digiti minimi	Pisiform to proximal phalanx of 5th digit	Flexes and abducts 5th digit	Ulnar (C8-T1)
Flexor digiti minimi	Flexor retinaculum and hamate to the proximal phalanx of the 5th digit	Flexes 5th digit	Ulnar (C8-T1)
Opponens digiti minimi	Hamate to the 5th metacarpal	Opposes 5th digit	
Palmaris brevis	Palmar aponeurosis to the skin of the hypothenar eminence	Tightens palmar aponeurosis	
First through fourth lumbricals	Tendons of flexor digitorum profundus to the medial 4 digits	Flex and extend medial 4 digits	Median (C5-T1) and ulnar (C8-T1)
First through fourth dorsal interossei	By two heads from the metacarpals to the proximal phalanx of the 2nd through 4th digits	Flexes and extends medial 4 digits	Ulnar (C8-T1)
First through third palmar interossei	Metacarpals 2, 4, and 5 to the proximal phalanx of those same digits	Flexes and extends digits	
Superficial flexor compartment of the forearm			
Pronator teres	Medial epicondyle of the humerus and coronoid process to the mid-lateral surface of the radius	Pronates forearm; flexes elbow	Median (C5-T1)
Flexor carpi radialis	Medial epicondyle of the humerus to the base of the 2nd metacarpal	Flexes and abducts wrist (palmaris longus also flexes elbow)	Median (C5-T1)
Palmaris longus	Medial epicondyle of the humerus to the palmar aponeurosis and flexor retinaculum		
Flexor carpi ulnaris	Medial epicondyle of the humerus and olecranon to the pisiform, hook of hamate, and 5th metacarpal	Flexes and adducts wrist	Ulnar (C8-T1)
Flexor digitorum superficialis	Medial epicondlye of the humerus, proximal ulna, and anterior radius to the phalanges of the medial 4 digits	Flexes medial 4 digits	Median (C5-T1)
Deep flexor compartment of the forearm			
Flexor digitorum profundus	Proximal, medial ulna and interosseous membrane to the distal phalanges of the medial 4 digits	Flexes wrist and medial 4 digits	Median (C5-T1) and ulnar (C8-T1)
Flexor pollicis longus	Anterior surface of the radius to the distal phalanx of the pollex	Flexes pollex	Median (C5-T1)

Muscle	Attachment Points	Action	Innervation
Pronator quadratus	Distal ulna to distal radius on their anterior surfaces	Pronates forearm	Median (C5-T1)
Neck			
Splenius (cervicis, capitis)	SPs of C3-T6 to the TPs of C1 and C2 and the mastoid process and nuchal line of the occiput	Bilaterally: extends cervical spine and head Unilaterally: sidebends and rotates the head ipsilaterally	Dorsal rami of the cervical spinal nerves
Semispinalis (thoracis, cervicis, capitis)	Occiput and SPs of cervical and dorsal spine to the TPs 2-4 segments inferior	Bilaterally: extends spine and head Unilaterally: sidebends and rotates spine	Dorsal rami of the spinal nerves from the surrounding segments
Longus (colli/cervicis and capitis)	Colli/cervicis: anterior bodies of C4-T3 to C2-C4 (vertical); TPs C3-C5 to anterior tubercle of C1 (superior oblique); TPs C5-C6 to anterior bodies of T1-T3 Capitis: TPs of C3-C6 to basilar part of occiput	Bilaterally: flexes head and cervical spine Unilaterally: sidebends and rotates head and neck ipsilaterally	Cervical spinal nerves and cervical plexus
Scalenes (anterior, middle, posterior)	Anterior: Anterior tubercles C3-C6 to rib 1 Middle: Posterior tubercles C2-C7 to rib 1 Posterior: Posterior tubercles C4-C6 to rib 2	Bilaterally: flexes neck Unilaterally; sidebends cervical spine ipsilaterally; raises ribs	Cervical spinal nerves and brachial plexus
Sternocleidomastoid	Mastoid process and nuchal line to the manubrium and clavicle	Bilaterally: extends head Unilaterally: sidebends head ipsilaterally and rotates head contra laterally	CNXI Spinal accessory (C1-C6) and cervical spinal nerves
Suboccipitals			
Rectus capitis posterior (major and minor)	Major: Nuchal line of occiput to SP of C2 Minor: Nuchal line of occiput to posterior tubercle of C1	Bilaterally: extends head Unilaterally: rotates head ipsilaterally	Dorsal rami of the suboccipital (C1) nerve
Rectus capitis anterior	Basilar part of occiput, anterior of occipital condyles, to lateral mass of C1	Bilaterally: flexes head Unilaterally: Sidebends head ipsilaterally	
Rectus capitis lateralis	Basilar part of occiput, lateral of occipital condyles, to lateral mass of C1		

Muscle	Attachment Points	Action	Innervation
Obliquus capitis (superior and inferior)	Superior: Nuchal line to TP of C1 Inferior: TP of C1 to SP of C2	Bilaterally: extends head Unilaterally: sidebends head ipsilaterally and rotates contralaterally (superior); rotates head ipsilaterally (inferior)	Dorsal rami of the suboccipital (C1) nerve
Infrahyoids			
Sternohyoid	Manubrium to hyoid	Depresses hyoid and larynx	Ansa cervicalis, inferior trunk (C1-C3)
Sternothyroid	Manubrium to thyroid cartilage		
Thyrohyoid	Thyroid cartilage to hyoid	Depresses hyoid and elevates larynx	
Omohyoid	Hyoid to superior border of the scapula via superior and inferior bellies	Depresses, retracts, and steadies hyoid	
Suprahyoids (Oral Diaphragm)			
Geniohyoid	Inferior mental spine of mandible to hyoid	Elevates and protracts hyoid	Ansa cervicalis
Mylohyoid	Mylohyoid line of mandible to hyoid	Elevates hyoid and floor of mouth	CNV3 Trigeminal (mandibular branch)
Stylohyoid	Styloid process of temporal bone to hyoid	Elevates and retracts hyoid	CNVII (facial)
Digastric	Digastric fossa of mandible (anterior belly) to the mastoid (posterior belly) via an intermediate tendon on the hyoid	Depresses mandible; raises hyoid during swallowing	CNV3 Trigeminal for anterior belly (mandibular branch) and CNVII Facial for posterior belly
Muscles of Mastication			
Medial pterygoid	Medial surface of lateral pterygoid plate and pterygoid fossa to medial surface of the ramus of mandible	Elevates mandible	CNV3 Trigeminal (mandibular branch)
Lateral pterygoid	Greater wing of the sphenoid (superior head) to TMJ capsule; lateral surface of lateral pterygoid plate (inferior head) to the condylar process of the mandible	Laterally deviates, elevates, and protrudes mandible	
Masseter	Zygomatic arch, anteriorly (superficial portion) and posteriorly (deep portion) to the ramus of the mandible	Elevates and protrudes mandible	
Temporalis	Temporal fossa to the coronoid process and ramus of mandible	Elevates and retracts mandible	

Muscle	Attachment Points	Action	Innervation
Extraocular muscles			
Superior levator palpebrae	Sphenoidal orbit to eyelid	Elevates and retracts eyelid	CNIII Oculomotor
Superior rectus	Common tendinous ring to superior/anterior surface of sclera	Adducts, depresses, and internally rotates eye	
Inferior rectus	Common tendinous ring to inferior/anterior surface of sclera	Depresses and adducts eye	
Medial rectus	Common tendinous ring to medial/anterior surface of sclera	Adducts and moves eye medially	
Lateral rectus	Common tendinous ring to lateral/anterior surface of sclera	Abducts eye laterally	CNVI Abducens
Superior oblique	Common tendinous ring to superior/lateral sclera via a tendinous portion that passes through a fibrocartilaginous ring	Medially rotates eye	CNIV Trochlear
Inferior oblique	Maxillary orbit to inferior lateral sclera	Laterally rotates eye	CNIII Oculomotor

References

Aalkaer, C., and Nilsson, H. (2005). Vasomotion: cellular background for the oscillator and for the synchronizationof smooth muscle cells. *British Journal of Pharmacology*, 144. 605-616.

Abbott, C.J., Choe, T.E., Burgoyne, C.F., Cull, G., Wang, L., and Fortune, B. (2014). Comparison of Retinal Nerve Fiber Layer Thickness In Vivo and Axonal Transport after Chronic Intraocular Pressure Elevation in Young versus Older Rats. *PLoS ONE*, 9 (12): e114546. doi:10.1371/journal.pone.0114546

Balaratnasingam, C., Morgan, W.H., Bass, L., Matich, G., Cringle, S.J., and Yu, D.Y. (2007). Axonal transport and cytoskeletal changes in the laminar regions after elevated intraocular pressure. *Investigative Ophthalmology & Visual Science*, 48 (8). 3632-3644.

Chalfie, M. (2009). Neurosensory mechanotransduction. *Nature Reviews Molecular Cell Biology*, 10. 44-52. doi:10.1038/nrm2595.

Disease. (n.d.). In *Merriam-Webster Medical*, an Encyclopaedia Brittanica Company online. Retrieved from http://www.merriam-webster.com/medical/disease

DuFort, C., Paszek, M.J., and Weaver, V.M. (2011). Balancing forces: architectural control of mechanotransduction. *Nature Reviews Molecular Cell Biology*, 12. 308-319. doi:10.1038/nrm3112.

Geiger, B., Spatz, J.P., and Bershadsky, A.D. (2009). Environmental sensing through focal adhesions. *Nature Reviews Molecular Cell Biology*, 10. 21-33. doi:10.1038/nrm2593.

Hahn, C., and Scwhartz, M.A. (2009). Mechanotransduction in vascular physiology and athereogenesis. *NatureReviews Molecular Cell Biology*, 10. 53-62. doi:10.1038/nrm2596.

Jaalouk, D.E., and Lammerding, J. (2009). Mechanotransduction gone awry. *Nature Reviews Molecular Cell Biology*, 10. 63-73. doi:10.1038/nrm2597.

Jaggar, J.H., Porter, V.A., Lederer, W.J., and Nelson, M.T. (2000). Calcium sparks in smooth muscle. *American Journalof Physiology and Cellular Physiology*, 278. 235-256.

Johnston, T.B., Davies, D.V., and Davies, F. (1958). *Gray's Anatomy 32nd Edition*. Toronto: Longmans, Green and Co.

Kuchera, M.L., and Kuchera, W.A. (1993). *Osteopathic Principles in Practice*. Dayton, Ohio: Greyden Press.

McConnell, C.P., and Teall, C.C. (1906). *The Practice of Osteopathy*. Kirksville, Missouri: The Journal Printing Co.

McLean, W.G. (1988). Pressure-induced inhibition of fast axonal transport of proteins in the rabbit vagus nerve in galactose neuropathy: prevention by an aldose reductase inhibitor. *Diabetologia*, 31 (7). 443-448.

Moore, K.L., Dalley, A.F., and Agur, A.M.R. (2014). *Clinically Oriented Anatomy 7th Edition*. Baltimore: Wolters Kluwer.

Parsons, J. (2006). *Osteopathy: Models for Diagnosis, Treatment, and Practice*. Toronto: Elsevier Limited.

Paulus, S. (n.d.). Expanding the Reach of Osteopathic Principles and Practice. In *An Introduction to the Analects of A.T. Still (24)*. Retrieved from http://osteopathichistory.com/pagesside2/Analects.html

Principles. (n.d.). In *Merriam-Webster,* an Encyclopaedia Brittanica Company online. Retrieved from http://www.merriam-webster.com/dictionary/principles

Quigley, H., and Anderson, D.R. (1976). The dynamics and location of axonal transport blockade by acute intraocularpressure elevation in primate optic nerve. *Investigative Ophthalmology*, 15 (8). 606-616.

Shirakashi, M. (1990). The effects of intraocular pressure elevation on optic nerve axonal transport in the monkey. *Acta ophthalmologica*, 68 (1). 37-43.

Still, A.T. (1897). *Autobiography of A.T. Still*. Kirksville, Missouri: Published by the author. eBook version: Inter Linea (June, 2004).

—. (1908). *Autobiography of Andrew T. Still*. Revised edition. Kirksville, Missouri: Published by the author.

—. (1910). *Osteopathy, Research and Practice*. Kirksville, Missouri: The Journal Printing Co. eBook version: Inter Linea (May, 2005).

—. (1902). *Philosophy and Mechanical Principles of Osteopathy*. Kansas City, MO: Hudson-Kimberly Publishing Company.

—. (1899). *Philosophy of Osteopathy*. Kirksville, MO: A.T. Still.

—. (1899). *Philosophy of Osteopathy*. Kirksville, Missouri: Published by the author. eBook version: Inter Linea (April, 2004).

Trowbridge, C. (2007). *Andrew Taylor Still, 1828-1917*. Kirksville, Missouri: Truman State University Press.

Schuenke, M., Schulte, E., and Schumacher, U. (2010). *Thieme Atlas of Anatomy*. New York: Thieme New York.

Wozniak, M.A., and Chen, S.C. (2009). Mechanotransduction in development: a growing role for contractility. *Nature Reviews Molecular Cell Biology*, 10. 34-43. doi:10.1038/nrm2592.

World Health Organization (2006). *Constitution of the World Health Organization*. Retrieved from http://www.who.int/governance/eb/who_constitution_en.pdf

Zink, G.J., and Lawson, W.B. (1979). An Osteopathic Structural Examination and Functional Inter-pretation of the Soma. *Osteopathic Annals*, 7, 12-19.

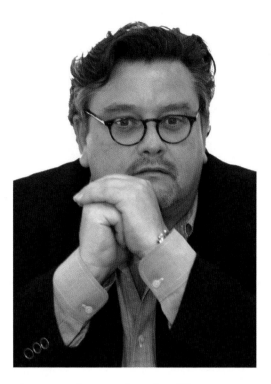

"I've always been passionate about instilling a new way of thinking in my classroom. Offering each student a unique learning experience tailored to their individual needs is a critical factor in establishing a successful educational program. Our course material isn't technique-driven or memorized from a textbook. It's designed to be hands-on, interactive, and really give students a legitimate understanding of human anatomy and physiology."

—Robert Johnston, CAO Principal

The faculty of the Canadian Academy of Osteopathy is headed by Robert Johnston. Mr. Johnston is Founder and Principal of the Canadian Academy of Osteopathy, and the Founder of both the Ontario Osteopathic Association, and the Canadian Institute of Classical Osteopathy. He is an enthusiastic and highly motivated clinical teacher and international lecturer who has dedicated his life to the promotion of Early American Classical Osteopathy. He has trained as a manual therapist in Canada, did his clinical internship in the United States, and trained directly under the late John Wernham in his post-graduate studies at the John Wernham College of Classical Osteopathy. Since then, it has been his goal to offer a progressive curriculum built on the proven theories and methodologies of Osteopathy's founding fathers. He continues to develop mechanical models for the student to approach osteopathic treatment. With ten years of experience as a clinical instructor and over twenty-five years of practice in manual therapy, Mr. Johnston possesses a rare talent for inspiring his students to reach the highest levels of academic performance.